MENOPAUSE WISDOMS

Women's Stories of Becoming Crone

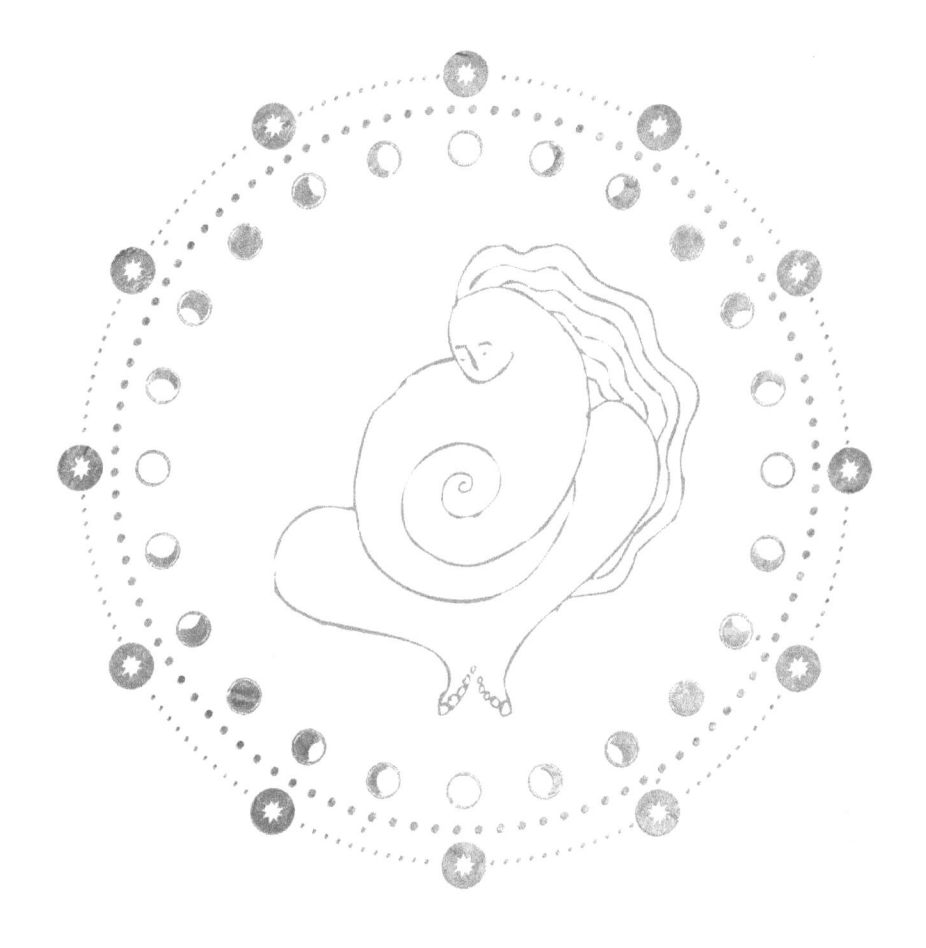

BRIER HEART

Copyright © 2022 by Brier Heart

All rights reserved. No part of this publication may be reproduced, distributed or transmitted in any form or by any means without permission of the publisher, except in the case of brief quotations referencing the body of work and in accordance with copyright law.

ISBN:

(Paperback) 978-1-913590-44-4

(ebook) 978-1-913590-45-1

Cover design by Lynda Mangoro

Goddess original art work by Carmen Friedman

The Unbound Press

www.theunboundpress.com

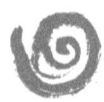

Hey unbound one!

Welcome to this magical book brought to you by The Unbound Press.

At The Unbound Press we believe that when women write freely from the fullest expression of who they are, it can't help but activate a feeling of deep connection and transformation in others. When we come together, we become more and we're changing the world, one book at a time!

This book has been carefully crafted by both the author and publisher with the intention of inspiring you to move ever more deeply into who you truly are.

We hope that this book helps you to connect with your Unbound Self and that you feel called to pass it on to others who want to live a more fully expressed life.

With much love,

Nicola Humber

Founder of The Unbound Press

www.theunboundpress.com

With love and gratitude to Cherilyn for bringing the Goddess, Women's Circle's and Moon Magic into my life.

CONTENTS

Welcome	9
Honouring My Sisters Poem	11
Introduction	13
The Language I Use	15
Part One: Changing the Narrative	17
Part Two: Becoming Crone	37
Exploring Women's Experiences of Menopause	39
Brier	43
Bev	65
Jenny	81
Louisa	101
Maggie	129
Meg	145
Mia	173
Nicola	191
Louise	211
Sharie	239
Sitali	255
Pearl	267

Part Three: Self-Care and Love	287
Exploring A New Perspective	289
Journey to Your Ancestors	291
Womb Meditation	294
Womb Moon Dance	296
Womb Healing and Womb Blessing	299
ReWilding with Nature	300
Cycles Chart	302
Deepen Your Connection with the Four Female Archetypes	305
Feminine and Masculine Energetic Qualities	307
Reclaiming Your Menarche Ritual	309
Feminine Rising Poem and Music	311
Dark Moon Dreaming	313
Creating an Altar to Honour Yourself as Crone	315
Further Exploration	316
Acknowledgements	318
About the Author	319

WELCOME

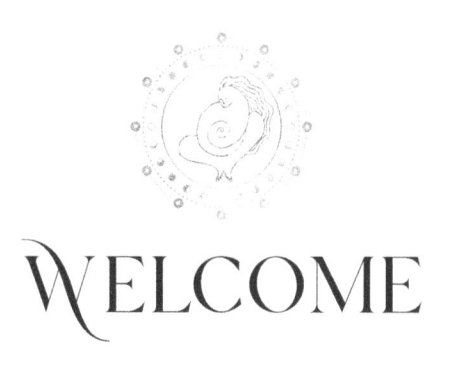

Dear Sister,

I am so happy to welcome you to *Menopause Wisdoms – Women's Stories of Becoming Crone*.

I embrace you with love and sisterhood in this moment of you choosing to step over the threshold into your isolation, death and rebirth, an initiation; that is the alchemy of menopause.

Know that in this moment, you are saying 'yes' to honouring the amazing woman you are, 'yes' to throwing off the shrouds of shaming and diminishing that we have been told we must wear as we become an elder.

I invite you to explore what it is to be a changing woman when we question the narrative of negativity and create one that welcomes, celebrates and values those changes as our gateway to becoming Crone – a potent and powerful Wild Wise Woman.

The journey these following pages will take you on, invites you to develop a new language and attitude towards your changing mind, body and spirit.

You will be walking a pathway to being who you want to be in the world as you learn a language of empowerment, awaken to your cyclical nature, your womb wisdom and to the beauty of becoming an elder.

So, dearest Sister, take a deep breath and let's begin………….

Honouring My Sisters

Let me hold space for you,
I am holding space for you.
I will witness you.
I will honour your courage.
My tears will fall and flow with yours.
You are not alone dearest one.
Look behind you, you will see them all –
Your sisters, your ancestors standing strong,
Hand in hand, in hand in hand.
Let us catch you, as you fall.
We are holding space
For your rage, your pain, your grief,
For your undoing, your searching, your discovering.
We will dance with you around the fire of your disintegration.
We will enter the cave with you and hear your wailing,
Your laughter and your joy.
We will lay naked with you,
As you crawl, rebirthing from the Earth.
You are reclaiming that which was stolen from you, my love.
You are rewilding the true nature of who you are.

Brier Heart

INTRODUCTION

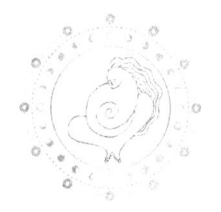

If we were sitting together at the kitchen table, right now, with a cup of tea and piece of cake, I'd love to ask you how you are feeling as you begin this exploration into Menopause Wisdoms. I wonder where you feel you are on your menopause journey? What are your experiences so far? Perhaps, you are struggling with your own and others' attitudes towards your transformation. Or maybe, you want to pack your suitcase and run for the hills to find solitude and quiet?

My hope is, that whatever you are experiencing, what you read in the following pages will support you, inform you and hold you within a loving container.

Menopause Wisdoms – Women's Stories of Becoming Crone, is set out in three parts.

In Part One, I share with you those things I have learnt from my own journey as well as those of the women I have facilitated to travel through their changes. I have a particular view that we have been mis-led all these years about what it is to be a menopausal woman. My perspective came from learning Self-Care and Love; through sitting in circle with other women, being in nature as much as I could be and from creating ritual and ceremony as I began to honour my changes, heal my wounding and commit to practices for my wellbeing. This did not come easily to begin with. It felt uncomfortable, alien, selfish and indulgent to put my own needs first. Over time, I learnt that the gift of Self-Care and Love was key to experiencing my menopausal years as an alchemical process.

In Part Two, you will read the stories of twelve women (including my own), telling you how they journeyed or are journeying through their changes. Their voices ring through with authenticity, courage, honour and love. There are three reflective questions repeated at the end of each story to support you in beginning to consider how you want to explore your own transformational journey. I have always enjoyed using a beautiful journal to record my thoughts, questions and insights as I venture through a book, programme, course and day to day life. I suggest you gift yourself one. It is, in itself, an act of honouring your commitment to making time and space for yourself to read the following. A journal is like a listening heart, a confidant, a space in which you can be truly yourself as you note down what emerges for you.

In Part Three, are ideas for creating your own pathways to Self-Care and Love. I share with you some of the practices I have used over the last ten years. These are suggestions, and certainly not intended as a prescription! I strongly believe in encouraging *your own* creativity, your own medicine. I consider my role to be a guide and facilitator. As a post-menopausal woman, I continue to find value in them and have learnt to adapt and change as and when my wisdom calls me to do so.

I trust that you will use this book in whatever way best suits you. You may choose to read it in the order it is set out; but as one changing woman to another, I highly recommend you give yourself permission to go with your flow and curiosity. Tune in to your intuition, feel into what is calling you, allow yourself to gently meander your way through, if that feels right or you may prefer to plunge into the rapids and surge your way through! It's all perfect.

I am deeply grateful to the weaving of magic we women co-create and that through our magic, you have found your way to this book. I have written the following with love and hope, that as we each find our way home to our true nature, we are creating spaciousness for birthing a new way of being on this beautiful planet, walking lightly with grace and gratitude.

I welcome your thoughts and curiosities about what you will shortly read. Do get in touch here at **www.spiralsofwellbeing.co.uk** if you'd like to have a chat.

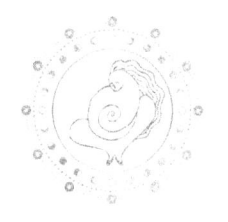

The Language I Use

Language is powerful. We know this from our learnt behaviours borne out of what we have been told we should be as a woman, especially as we become an older woman. How many times have you heard a menopausal woman being referred to in a derogatory way? Her hot flashes or forgetfulness being ridiculed? Her alchemical transformation being diminished and controlled?

Throughout the following pages I have strived to use a language of empowerment, celebration, respect, love and honouring of our menopausal changes.

The following is a list of the language I use.

The Menopause: The whole experience. Encompassing the phases, symptoms, changes, transformation.

Initiation: The Menopause

Isolation Phase: Perimenopause

Death Phase: Menopause

Rebirth: Post-menopause

Womb: When I refer to the womb, I am referring to the energy centre and, if you have a womb, the physical organ too. If you no longer have a physical womb, your womb energy remains. This continues to be your centre of creativity. It is also where your sacral chakra energy flows, a source of pleasure and desire.

Rewild/Wilding: To awaken and connect to your intuition, instinct and innate wisdom. When you feel the desire to dance to the rhythm of Mother Earth's energy and hear the song of your Soul.

Alchemy: The power and process of change and transformation, in a magical and potent way.

Menarche: The start of menstruation.

Yoni: Your vagina, labia, vulva, clitoris, cervix, womb, ovaries.

Waxing Moon: Any-time after the dark/new moon and before the full moon.

Waning Moon: Any-time after the full moon and before the dark/new moon.

Wild Wise Woman: A woman awakened and connected to her cyclical nature, her intuition, instinct, potency and power and to the loving energy of nature and Mother Earth.

Elder: A wise woman of any age who holds space and counsel for others within a tribe or other group.

Sacred: Dedicated to a purpose of value and importance to you.

Ritual: An action which serves as a bridge between our outer and inner worlds and between the ordinary and the extraordinary.

The Four Female Archetypes: Maiden. Mother. Enchantress. Crone. See page 302 Cycles Chart.

Masculine/Feminine Energetic Qualities: See page 307.

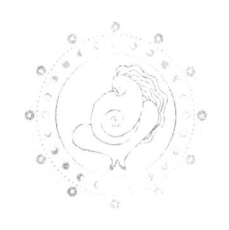

Part One
Changing the Narrative

The Menopause has been sold to us as a negative phase of our lives for way too long. We have been fed the lie that when we reach our menopausal years we become 'less than,' 'crazy,' 'embarrassing,' 'irrational,' 'too much' to be around. We have been taught that our menopausal symptoms need to be got rid of, controlled at all cost and are regarded always as an inconvenience.

It is little wonder then, that many of us are fearful of The Menopause.

That we fight against our hot flushes, our greying hair, our changing body, our feelings of loss, of grief and of rage.

That many of us feel diminished, invisible, lost and alone.

It is time then to change the narrative.

Time for the negative perceptions, messages and images we have been taught and shown, to be dispelled.

Time to speak about our changes openly and with respect, grace and honesty.

I am here to let you know that actually, our menopausal years are an invitation to us to step into our authority, our potency and our power.

There was a time, long, long ago when we lived to the rhythm of our own and nature's cycles. Our menstrual blood was sacred. A woman would give her menstrual blood to the land she inhabited, to nurture and nourish the herbs and food she grew – just as she was then nurtured and nourished by her labours. Her relationship with her menstrual and life cycle, nature and the phases of the moon was a dance to the heart beat of her Soul and of Mother Earth.

In every village there was a wise woman. She was a midwife, a herbalist, a healer, a shaman, a witch, a crone. She was revered, honoured and respected.

And then came patriarchy.

The loving power of women, our feminine energy, was a threat to the agenda of patriarchal control and greed.

The Inquisitions and witch hunts over hundreds of years were responsible for the murders of tens of thousands of women whose only crime was to be female in a patriarchal world. We were imprisoned, raped, tortured, drowned and burnt at the stake, if we dared to share or express our potency. If we managed to survive, we were shunned from our communities, friends and family.

We learned to keep our magic hidden.

We learned to be fearful of our innate wisdom.

Men and women were taught to mistrust each other. Women were turned against women. Communities became divided and slowly but surely, we became disconnected from our intuition and from the song of our Soul.

Our menstrual blood became shameful.

Our desires and pleasures were sinful.

To be a woman was dangerous.

To be a Wild Wise Woman, a Crone, became a subject of derision. We were portrayed as withered, ugly, unkind, even evil. If you look up the definition of Crone in a dictionary it says, 'An ugly, malicious old woman.'

The legacy of being demonised all those centuries ago clearly perpetuates, even today in the 21st century. The view that, to be a post-menopausal woman, a Crone, still signifies being that ugly, malicious old woman. And it may be that you have felt a contraction each time I've used the word Crone. It is hardly surprising if you did. The patriarchy has done a very good job in demonising the power of women elders. We carry in our cells the knowledge that our ancestors were put to death for their natural potency.

So, let's get this sorted now, because I use the word Crone a lot!

Crone actually means a wise woman. As simple as that. She is the archetype that represents rebirth, worldliness, compassion, authority, potency, power, grace.

Sadly, most of us have never been told this!

So, it probably comes as no surprise that we lost the thread to our ancestral wisdom, we lost our Wildness and our connection to our cyclical energy, we lost our link to the true nature of who we are.

But we are rising again!

The voices of our ancestors are calling to us:

"Rise up sisters, rise up."

We are reclaiming what was taken from us.

We are walking out from the flames.

We are gathering our bones.

We are coming home to our feminine power.

And, let us be very clear about our power.

The power I am speaking of is not power over others – we do not want to become the corruptors. It is rather, having an ability to be response-able, to be in our own authority, to choose for ourselves, to be grounded, present and clear.

So, let's take a few breaths all the way down into the beautiful darkness of our womb where we *remember* there is magic in being a (menopausal) woman.

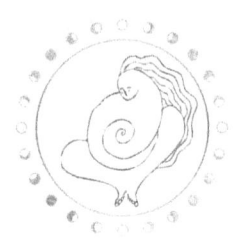

We women are cyclical beings, you know this, I'm sure. But how many of us are or were attuned to our menstrual cycle? How many of us are aware of our daily rhythms, to the phases of the moon, to natures cycles, let alone to our life cycle?

Knowing our cycle and developing a deep connection to it, whether it be our menstrual cycle (which may already be irregular or stopped altogether), our life cycle, natures cycles and the moon phases, allows us to make choices aligned to our needs and desires as they flow and fluctuate throughout our changes.

During our menopausal years we can feel adrift as we lose connection to our menstrual cycle, no longer able to chart our familiar rhythms. That is, if we *had* a connection to our cycle, if we *did* chart and if our cycle was *familiar* to us. Often, many of us have gone through our menstruating years disconnected from our womb and our changing rhythms each month.

How does being connected to our cyclical rhythms help us?

Charting our unique rhythms helps us to know when we are at our most creative, or when our energy tends to be low, when we want to be alone or when we want to be around others. We can plan our work and leisure schedules in response to our cyclical wisdom. We can learn to communicate our needs, to take responsibility for expressing what we need and want. During our menopausal years, our ability to do this is imperative to our wellbeing and as we lose our menstrual cycle, it is ever more important to be attuned to nature's and the moon cycles.

When we become aligned not only to our female cycles, but also to the cycles of nature and the moon, we begin to notice our shifting energies more acutely. We open ourselves to the gifts each season and each moon phase offers us. We become more deeply connected to our innate intuition and instinct, to Mother Earth and therefore to our true nature. This knowledge, this alignment, supports us throughout our changes.

I remember when I was pregnant (many moons ago!) how utterly exhausted I was in the first and last trimesters. I didn't experience that type of exhaustion again until I was menopausal. Fortunately, I had already learnt that to ignore my body, mind, spirit callings were detrimental to my wellbeing. I had learnt to listen and respond with kindness and love to my needs.

But for many of us this is not so.

As it was during our menstruating years to be told, 'Just get on with it,' the attitude towards The Menopause is to, 'Put on a brave face.' We are not encouraged or supported to recognise our changes as messages of wisdom and of our need to be held with loving kindness.

The Menopause, an initiation, however, *demands* that we pay attention to our needs. If we do not, we live with the consequences of perpetuating those negative attitudes and experiences we are working to re-write together.

As we lose the thread of our menstrual cycle, we enter a phase of not knowing. When will I bleed next? Will I bleed again? How heavy will the blood flow be? Will this bleeding ever stop?

But our cyclical nature does not go away because we stop menstruating. We become *more* aware of our life cycle, of stepping over the threshold into our isolation, death and rebirth, the initiation through which we become crone.

Because we may not have consciously connected to being cyclical, bit by bit we lost ease of access to our intuition and to the rhythm of our own dance, thereby forgetting the true nature of who we are. But what we forget can be re-membered as we walk a path of rewilding.

A woman who no longer menstruates, whose place in the world is nudged and poked and rattled by negative attitudes and perceptions; carries in her bones and deep within her Soul a longing for rewilding.

The calling of our initiation, if we choose to listen more deeply is:

"Go inward and seek all that you have ignored, buried or denied. Acknowledge what no longer serves you. Listen deeply to your inner wisdom. Welcome back your Wild Wise Woman self into your bones."

It is time to re-member; heal and honour the amazing woman you have always been.

What difference does it make to re-member what we lost and forgot in relation to being cyclical? Why does being awakened to our cyclical nature and the true nature of who we are make a difference to our lives?

Quite simply the differences are life changing.

We re-wild ourselves.

We come home to ourselves.

We set ourselves free.

We make choices aligned to who we truly are.

Our transformation offers us an opportunity to be the ones who make the changes our world so desperately needs. By reclaiming our initiation, as the alchemical process it has always been, we are re-igniting the flame of our potency and power to illuminate the *magic* of being a woman as we become an elder. We are helping to heal ancestral pain and our lineage. We are forgiving our mothers who did not know how to heal and so, unknowingly, perpetuated the myth that women are on a downward spiral once they reach The Menopause.

Why did our mothers not know how to heal their wounding?

Why do so many of us continue to struggle with being menopausal and reach for medical intervention as a first or only option?

I have no doubt that the answers lie in us still living in a patriarchal world which regards our changes as an embarrassment and something to be contained. The Menopause has been medicalised. Menopausal women have been marginalised by these negative attitudes and behaviours which seek to devalue this phase of our lives.

Patriarchy has created a masculine heavy energy world which is predominantly linear, rational, analytical. There is of course nothing inherently wrong with those qualities. However, when they are not balanced with feminine energy qualities such as vision, reflection, compassion and flow we end up fearful of feeling deeply, our creativity becomes blocked, any flicker of intuitive expression is shut down.

Trying to maintain a linear and rational perspective of life creates havoc for a changing woman. When we begin to feel the undoing of ourselves during our transformation, the rational masculine energy gets in the way of our intuitive feminine energy. A hot flush becomes irritating or unbearable, when it could be experienced as a powerful cleansing. Insomnia becomes a wakeful nightmare, exhausting and unacceptable, when it could be a time of quiet reflection, an opportunity to be still and silent with no interruptions. Exhaustion prevents us from concentrating and working to our typical busy schedules, when it could be used as a signal to prioritise differently, learning to attune to our new rhythms.

We are not taught that our 'symptoms' are actually messages from our mind, body and spirit, offering pathways to shedding what no longer serves us in order to transform into The Wild Wise Woman we long to be.

There is no denying that the way our society is structured, the systems in which we all have to find a way to function, are not Menopause friendly. We are required to care for our children (the onset of our changes occurs for women of all ages), our parents, and our home in addition to having a full-time job, part-time job, more than one job, no job. Life is demanding and we are rarely taught or shown that rest, slowing down, dare I say, even stopping our frenzied multi-tasking, is okay. We are often not offered any support. We rarely ask for it, believing we are failing if we do or that we are unworthy of help.

For me this is the real problem. We live in a world that values 'doing.' We have come to believe that if we are not 'doing' we are not valuable. We must carry on producing at all costs.

At all costs.

The cost for us as (menopausal) women is often depletion and depression. We have not been empowered or enabled to create space in which to approach our changes as a *gift* rather than something to be controlled.

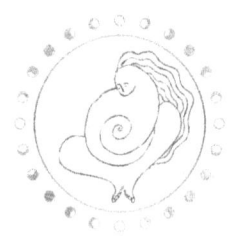

The Menopause calls us to look at all our unspoken wounding, which often invites our rage to be expressed. But we have been told rage is undesirable and unacceptable. We have been taught since childhood that being a 'good girl,' a quiet, compliant girl is required of us always. Our response to rage or exhaustion within this container pushes us to medicate our symptoms.

Yes, rage can be uncomfortable, yes it can be unpleasant and perhaps even scary but holding on to our wounding is detrimental to our wellbeing. Therefore, finding a safe container in which to express our rage, to be witnessed, to be held in love and compassion as we explore our grief and loss, we are empowering ourselves to heal. We begin to re-member ourselves, shedding what is not ours and never has been.

The world is changing. The Menopause is being talked about in the mainstream media (although sadly, often in medicalised language and attitude). Feminine energy is rising to address the imbalance of our current way of existing. We are learning to release ourselves from the bindings our mothers and grandmothers were not able to, being still shackled within a male, masculine energy heavy world.

While we rise up to create a new way of being on Earth, birthing a balance of the feminine and the masculine energy, in both women and men, there is much we can do to change the narrative. To travel our menopausal years differently to those generations of women who came before us, even within the restrictions of our current unbalanced and erratic world, is not only imperative for us but for all women who come after us.

When we realise that it is the attitudes and behaviours towards our transformation that need to change, we free ourselves to find ways in which to honour and embrace all of what that liberation brings. We free ourselves to take responsibility for our mind, body and spirit wellbeing.

For around three to four years, I didn't realise I was entering my menopausal years, I had been given zero information about what to expect. Not knowing, resulted in me having a rough time of it during those years. I had anxiety, palpitations, insomnia, depression and rage. Even when my body was screaming at me 'you're beginning your transformation!' with period pain like I hadn't experienced since my teenage years, the penny didn't drop. And why would it have done? I'd never been taught or told what to expect. No-one was talking about The Menopause; it was taboo to broach the subject. It felt lonely and confusing.

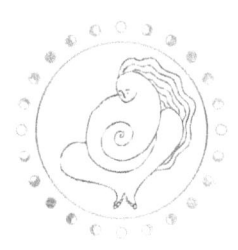

When I eventually found the courage to explore why my bleeding had become so heavy and painful and why I was needing to pee frequently, I was diagnosed with a uterine fibroid. I was offered a hysterectomy (surgically removing the womb and sometimes also the ovaries). Every time I went to have a routine scan, I was offered a hysterectomy. I was no longer in pain, the heavy bleeding I experienced had ceased. I was told the uterine fibroid posed no danger to me, and yet, I was asked if I wanted to have my womb removed!

Did you know there are around ten million women (in the UK) going through The Menopause, with you, right now? So why is it that what is on offer to us remains largely to do with treating our changes as an illness. We have known for a very long time that HRT (Hormone Replacement Therapy) and anti-depressants, which are prescribed to suppress our symptoms, carry risks to our health from mild, short-term effects to severe, life changing disease. And as it was in my case, many of us are often offered or advised to have a hysterectomy.

I am outraged that still, in the 21st Century, women continue to experience intrusive, often unnecessary, medical interventions as a *first* or *only* option.

In the USA, caesarean sections are more commonplace than natural births.

Here in the UK, mammograms are routine. In my experience they are often painful and I believe carry some risk. We are not informed of or given options for investigations and monitoring (unless we specifically request them) such as thermal imaging and/or ultra sound.

Pharmaceuticals are given to alleviate painful menstruation and menopausal symptoms without exploring, for example, a change of diet, exercise, herbal medicines, natural therapies. (See Susun S. Weed's book *Menopausal Years: The Wise Woman Way*).

It is of course sometimes necessary, even life-saving to undergo medical interventions. I have two friends who tried many different approaches and treatments to end their painful and debilitating heavy bleeding. For them both, in the end they had no other option than to have a hysterectomy. In these cases, it is vitally important to have pathways to and practices of Self-Care and Love for recovery and healing.

The medicalisation of our natural female changes has taught us to mistrust our intuition, our dreams and insights. We have lost our instinct, our innate ability to listen to the messages our bodies give us, to pay attention and be curious about the myriad of ways we can heal ourselves.

We have come to rely on the opinion of our GP (General Practitioner), consultants and other medical practitioners as our *only* source of information and treatment, and who typically respond to our changes as problems to be medicated.

Therefore, it follows that the messages we are given about The Menopause, continue to be diminishing and damaging to us.

I don't want that to be my daughter's experience, or your experience. I don't want any woman to enter her menopausal years blindfolded, gagged and in fear of what is actually a thread to her wisdom.

I feel empowered when I research procedures and treatments. I question, I go inward and connect with my innate wisdom, I take my time before making my choice. I am not saying this is easy to do, in my experience we (women) have not been shown, taught or encouraged to believe in our internal authority. I speak more of this later.

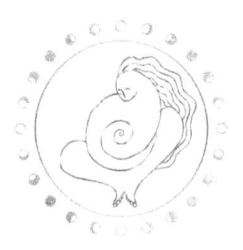

The Menopause has three distinct phases, isolation (perimenopause), death (menopause) and rebirth (post-menopause). These phases are our *initiation* to becoming Crone. Within each phase we experience our transformation at a mind and spirit level, and a transmutation at body level.

Understanding what may occur during the different phases of our initiation and how we can choose to interpret them, is worth exploring! It will make a significant, even profound difference to how you live and experience this alchemical journey.

We will each encounter the different phases of our changes in our own unique way, including how long each phase lasts and what happens within each phase.

So, I think it is helpful for you to know that your experience will unfold at your own pace and in your own way.

While writing this book, I have increasingly felt that the labels perimenopause, menopause and post-menopause tend to tie us up in knots, provoking us to continuously focus on the question, 'Which one am I?'

I recently invited the women in my Menopause Wisdoms Online Circle, as we moved into the soundscape meditation, to ask themselves the question:

'What would it feel like for me to let go of those labels and allow myself to *be* fully in what I am feeling?'

With their permission, here is what came through for Ali, Jane and Meg.

Ali: Initially I was taken by a sense of reluctant surprise. "Wait," I thought, "Haven't I been trying to claim this label of perimenopause and be more out and open with it through my language as a kind of 'owning'? Do I want to let that go?"

As I opened to the enquiry, though, I became aware of how delicious it might be to be free of the judgements, expectations and assumptions – my own and other people's that those labels invite in. Aren't most labels about simplifying, stereotyping and compartmentalising? A convenient way to sort, control, edit and process that make it too easy to ignore, diminish or dismiss the subtleties and differences of individual lived experience?

I'm left with the possibility that I can try just being with my experience from day to day, month to month with less of the judgements and assumptions brought about by labelling.

To sit with and express my experience in the present and from the fullness of my whole unlabelled being feels potent and welcome. It's something I will work with now and see where it takes me. At the very least I think I will be more discerning about when, why and by whom I allow this transitional life experience to be labelled.

Water was with me during the meditation. First, I was dancing – skimming almost – across a beach of fine sand. The gentle ebb and flow of waves provided a rhythm to move to inside and out and I had a sense of joy, lightness and freedom.

In moments I was floating – limbs splayed in a star shape – in a pool of still, dark water. I felt weightless, relaxed and at ease; fully supported. As I reflect now, this seems like an invitation to let go and allow myself to be held. Seaweed feels like a perfect symbol; anchored but floating in the current of whatever is present in any moment, on any day.

Jane: As I sat, I found myself on a beach, looking at the tide as it came in and out, and felt the pull of the moon creating a rhythm of life, and I realised that my body/I have been the 'tide' for 40 years now (since starting my bleeds), which seems an incredibly long time.

Remembering the question you set us, I thought that 'ebb and flow' was perhaps a good way to describe the sense of perimenopause, giving a less static terminology and sense than perimenopause, menopause, and post-menopause. However, I suddenly felt really sad that I may have had my last bleed now, and felt really unsettled and upset that the rhythm (the ebb and flow) my body was so used to was going to go, and I had no choice. It felt as though I'd need a period of mourning to cope with the loss…It felt like the pull of the moon, and the ebb and flow of the tides were being taken from me, in an enforced way, and that I wasn't ready for that; that I hadn't appreciated it enough somehow, while I had it.

Thinking back to the tides, I realised that if the tides stopped coming in and out, the effect would cause the world to tip into firstly impending chaos, and then chaos, and realised that maybe that's why perimenopause and menopause feel like impending chaos inside us. I felt anxious, as though I was in a state of impending chaos, and in the process of being cut out of the workings of the world – I didn't like it at all, especially that I had no choice, and that it was suddenly upon me...I felt a need to try and fix it; maybe I could keep my bleeds going longer with the right nutrition I told myself.

Within moments, remembering that years ago I had been a fixer, and had to learn to not try to fix things for people, I had the realisation that I don't need to fix it for myself either, but that I just needed to 'sit' with it. (I remember having the surprising side thought that this meditation, and the realisations I was having, felt like deep spiritual counselling coming from somewhere.)

As I then 'sat' with it, I watched the edge of the sea as it came in and out, and was aware at a deep level of all the many creatures in the beach and ocean habitats who had to live their lives being swept back and forth, or burying themselves to stay safe until the next tide, and coming up when they could... and I suddenly felt the constant relentlessness of the movement back and forth over me, as if I were one of the creatures dictated to for my survival by the tide, the water, and I desperately wanted the stillness that would come from not having to witness/be part of the constant movement.

I reflected that these days, my preferred spots for swimming are Llyns or lakes, and not the sea, and if possible at sunset...perhaps I am just catching up with what my body has been trying to show me for the last couple of years about what I need – swimming free and gently in calm still water, as I watch the sun set over the mountains; no longer buffeted by being dictated to, or the restlessness of lack of wisdom of earlier years... and I smiled, and it all felt OK, more than OK, good.

Meg: Rest. Deep rest. Relaxation. Campfire at night – darkness as comfort. COMFORT, rest. Present and still and quiet – drawn to the flame. Flame as agent of change. Watching the wood burn, glow, heat – feel the heat. Crumble. Mint plants – smell of fresh mint. Intoxicating. (Mint spreads like wildfire)

Ali, Jane and Meg clearly express how powerful an enquiry can be in supporting our transformation.

I have no doubt that the name we give to each phase is of less importance than how we approach and experience each of those phases.

My suggestion is that you take note of what you are feeling, of what is changing and rather than becoming anxious about where you are precisely on your journey, bring focus to Self Care and Love practices.

It will all unfold as it needs to.

The following descriptions are then what *typically* happens in each phase. But let us not forget, as a woman, our energy flows as it needs to flow when we attune ourselves to this alchemical process, so what changes, how and when, will be your own story, in your own time.

Phase One. Your initiation begins, this is the phase of isolation. Generally called perimenopause. These are the years when your menstrual cycle becomes irregular, you may have heavier bleeding but it can also be lighter. Often pre-menstrual tension may become heightened. You may have spotting or flooding. You are likely to be noticing something important is unfolding. Within your fluctuating, irregular cycle you may notice strong feelings emerging such as anger, bewilderment, sadness and a deep longing for isolation.

This is the tornado approaching!

You may feel trapped, yearning to be alone, to run away, to shut everyone else out. Your physical symptoms, such as hot flushes, insomnia, night sweats, palpitations, anxiety or exhaustion demand your attention. You are likely to have feelings of disintegration, of not knowing yourself, and having no control.

Your emotions may sway from utter blissfulness to screaming rage. Tears may flow at the sight of a beautiful flower, confusion or despair may consume you from hearing news of the world in crisis.

Let's not deny or pretend then, that our initiation is a walk in the park, it is not helpful for us to do so. In fact, to deny or pretend, is what we have been told we *should* do. The things I have described are our awakenings the patriarchy has led us to believe we must control, subdue and diminish at all costs.

These demands of the isolation phase are the beginning of our fragmentation, of unravelling all we think we know of ourselves. As we peel back our layers of protection and distraction, our disguises and false beliefs; all that we thought we knew, falls away.

Perceiving our disintegration as the letting go of, the process of healing our wounding, of seeing it is our gateway to gathering those pieces of our self that have been buried deep inside waiting to be freed, is the process of rewilding our true nature.

While it may feel incredibly uncomfortable to experience the range of mind, body, spirit challenges and awakenings, know that through this phase you are moving ever closer to becoming Crone, your Wild Wise Woman.

Phase Two. Meno (menstruation) pause (stops). This is the end of your menstrual flow. You may feel waves of grief and loss once your blood has finally stopped flowing. This is the death phase.

Menopause is indeed an ending, but *not* in the sense that our lives are over! It most certainly is a *death* experience *and* it is also a *rebirth* experience.

The alchemy of menopause is that we are undergoing a glorious transformation.

The tornado is passing!

Through the following fourteen moon cycles after your final bleed (at which point it is generally considered we become a post-menopausal woman), you will discover that in the centre of the tornado there is stillness, a place where we can begin to re-assemble ourselves, without all the clutter.

We are now reclaiming the knowledge that our symptoms are actually our pathways to healing our wounding in preparation for our new way of being, as we find our way home.

Having the courage to reshape and reclaim the sacredness and alchemy of being a changing woman and becoming Crone is a conscious act of the feminine rising. Being in our Truth, retelling *his*tory to *her*story, reshaping our experiences, showing up as we truly are, will slowly but surely, dismantle the old, worn out, destructive attitudes and behaviours towards this most amazing initiation.

The invitation is to dive deep, to welcome your vulnerability and be courageous.

Through my isolation and death phases, I learnt to enjoy diving into the darkness, a place that for many years felt unsafe to go. Because we are reclaiming our Wild Wise Woman self, we also need to reclaim the darkness. Just like our menstrual blood was demonised, so too has the darkness. We are taught as children to be afraid of the dark. We are told scary, dangerous creatures lurk in the shadows. As women, we have cause to be fearful of dark alleyways and streets, where there is potentially real danger. The dark has therefore become something which represents somewhere we should not venture.

We have been told that it is the 'light' where we will find our answers and comfort and therefore our happiness. Whilst the light is a source of wisdom, and it also nourishes and nurtures us, it sustains all life; it is important to remember that all living things come from the dark. Without the dark there would be no life.

We need the dark in which to rest and dream. The darkness reveals the stars and the moon. We see glowing, dancing firelight in the dark.

I have heard many people say of the dark:

"Oh, you don't want to go there!"

But actually, the dark, our *internal* place of darkness, is exactly where we need to go, in order to reveal and release our own stars and moon.

During your isolation phase, you will have been called into the dark, longing to be alone, undisturbed. As you entered your 'cave of solitude' you knew in your bones it was time to open your arms and heart and welcome the beautiful, life-giving dark.

During your death phase, when your blood cycle has ceased, you will feel a shift in energy. You will learn your cave of darkness is a place of rebirth. This phase invites you to prepare for your rebirth as an elder, re-integrating into the world.

It makes sense then, that connecting with your *womb* is a beautiful place in which to reclaim the dark in order to emerge reborn.

Your womb has guided you every month for many years within your menstrual cycle. At your time of pre-menstruation and menstruation, there was an invitation to go inward, down into the darkness. Your Enchantress energy has been within you always, coaxing you to find your edge, connect to your thunder, to explore your shadows. And just as you travelled through the darkness of pre-menstruation and menstruation to emerge back out into Spring (Maiden energy) and Summer (Mother energy) so you will too from your isolation and death phases, as you continue to walk your pathway to becoming Crone.

And remember always, that although this space of darkness may challenge us, we are reborn as a woman who has come back to herself, who has journeyed through her dissolution, has become adept at creating practices of Self-Care and Love and stands in her majesty. This is the alchemy – when we allow it to be.

Phase Three. Post-menopause is your rebirth and re-integration into the world. You step out of your cave.

Your healing pathways will have led you to feeling more deeply connected to yourself than ever before. You will be able to set boundaries with clarity and compassion for yourself and others. Your creativity and passion for life is boundless. How you move and speak and listen will be grounded in your deep wisdom. You will have learnt how to manage your time in relation to your energy and in relationship with the moon, seasons and your own daily cycles.

Your rebirth signifies the culmination of all you have learnt, all you have healed throughout your disintegration and re-membering. You are walking towards becoming Crone, a woman ready to stand in her potency, to bring to the world the gift of all that she is.

So, how do we manage all these changes throughout our initiation within the context of our day to day lives?

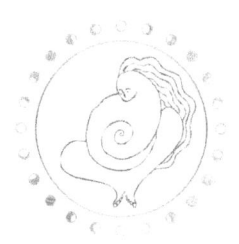

Finding your own healing pathways will be part of the process of your empowerment, of coming home to yourself. You will read, in Part Two, the stories of twelve women, each of whom share with you her struggles, her insights, her celebrations and how she discovered and created her own wellbeing practices. What you will discover through their shared wisdom, are pieces of gold, threads of magic, Wild Wise Women knowing, all of which will help you to navigate your journey.

There are also a number of practices I used and continue to use, shared in Part Three, Self-Care and Love. Being in sisterhood and nature, being heard and witnessed by other women was powerfully healing. Within that container I became friends with my cyclical nature, I attuned myself to the moon phases as I began to lose my menstrual cycle. Being in nature, held by the energy of trees, water, sky, birds, stillness, dark and light, was sacred medicine for me. Sisterhood and nature awakened my ability to consciously embrace wellbeing practices aligned to the song of my Soul and to the loving nature of Mother Earth.

The good news is, creating practices for wellbeing and healing is not rocket science. It is not complicated but it does take effort and commitment.

It requires us to learn how to cherish and support ourselves, not as occasional treats, which suggests something special, but as an essential part of our lives.

Knowing what we need and want is critically important throughout our transformation.

We need to know, that when we are exhausted, we must rest!

When we want to be alone, we need to create the space and time to be alone.

We need to pace ourselves to our changing rhythm in the world.

We need to be honest with ourselves, our friends and with our loved ones.

They too may find our changes challenging as we become more able to speak our Truth and to set our boundaries.

We need to be clear and compassionate as we learn to express ourselves in new ways.

The following twelve stories will provide you with insights into how you may experience your changes and how you may create what you need and want to support you on this most magnificent and magical journey.

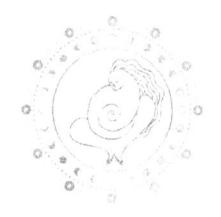

Part Two
Becoming Crone

In October 2019, my first book, *Take Off Your Armour and Have a Cup of Tea* was published. In this book I speak about being a mother of a child who shows up differently in the world and the magic she has brought to my life, in part, enabling me to embrace The Menopause as a deeply healing and alchemical process. As my book began to flow out into the world, I had a strong feeling that, what I had written about my own menopausal journey was just a beginning.

I travelled my menopausal years with other women in a loving, held space. We sat in circle together each month and explored what was calling us to dive into. I was curious. I allowed myself to be vulnerable. I was courageous, often confused, as layers of old patterning began to reveal itself to me. The container of the circle, the sisterhood, being heard, the processes and practices I learnt, guided me with tenderness through the challenges change inevitably brings. I opened myself to welcome, embrace and celebrate my transformation to becoming Crone.

I knew my experience was not typical. I knew the attitudes and behaviours towards and of menopausal women was still greatly shrouded in fear and shame. I felt in my bones it was time to clear away the hostility and negativity we and society hold in relation to the natural power of women; that is our innate cyclical wisdom, our blood, our creativity and our vigour as Crone.

I wanted to give space for other women to have their voices heard. I knew I needed to provide a held space for the women, just as I had been, and to create spaciousness for them to tell their story.

I decided to invite eleven women friends to contribute their individual, unique experiences of being menopausal. In the first instance, I explained my intention for the book and asked them to be interviewed. I then emailed them the following information. I based my prompts and questions on my personal experiences, knowledge and understanding of our initiation. Each prompt and question reflects the insights, learning and revelations I encountered during my transitions and ultimate transformation.

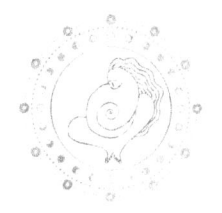

Exploring Women's Experiences of Menopause

Dearest Friend,

As you now know, I have decided to start my second book. A seed was planted on completion of 'Take off Your Armour and Have a Cup of Tea,' and I now feel ready to bring the message of reclaiming becoming Crone as an alchemical process.

I am so thrilled you are to be a part of this. I am beyond excited to provide an opportunity for your voice to be heard.

I believe by sharing your unique exploration and understanding of your changes you will bring profound healing for the women who read your words.

I believe too that the process I am inviting you to dive into offers you an opportunity to heal from generations of patriarchal wounding that has diminished us and swathed us in dishonour for being a woman, particularly a menopausal woman.

Before you look at the following prompts, please take a few moments to connect with your inner sense. You may like to create space and time for yourself, uninterrupted. Have a journal and a pen ready to make some notes.

Perhaps light a candle, lie or sit comfortably. Play some gentle music.

Close your eyes and take a few minutes to focus on your breath, allowing it to deepen and to fill your womb centre (below your belly and above your pubic bone) and yoni (your vagina, labia, vulva, clitoris).

When you feel ready, consciously, and silently in your head, say, "Hello," to your womb centre and yoni.

Continue to breathe deeply to your own rhythm, staying in connection to your womb centre and yoni. Stay in this place for 5 –10 minutes, or for however long feels good for you.

When you are ready, allow your breath to return to its usual pace, begin to wiggle your fingers and toes, have a stretch and a yawn, open your eyes.

Note down in your journal any feelings, memories, questions, sensations or anything else that came to you.

Put your journal to one side and take a look at the following prompts.

I suggest you take time for each one and record your response when you are ready in your journal.

Try not to censor what comes through! Allow your thoughts and feelings to flow, knowing that whatever arises is valid, worthy and wise.

- What have you been told or taught about what it is to be a woman? Think back to the first messages you were given from your mother, father, friends, media.
- How do you think those messages impacted on you as you transitioned from girl to woman?
- What are your memories of your menarche (first bleed)? How has that experience shaped your life as a woman? How has the experience of your first bleed impacted on you in relation to The Menopause?
- Did you know what to expect as you began your transition into your menopausal years?
- What messages were you given about The Menopause? Can you recall your mother's experience?
- Have there, are there aspects of The Menopause that you have enjoyed?
- Have there, are there aspects of The Menopause that you dislike?
- When you look in the mirror (if you do) what do you see?

- *What are your feelings about sex and your sexuality as a menopausal woman?*
- *Do you feel connected to your womb energy?*
- *Do you feel connected to your yoni energy?*
- *How do you feel about being a woman now you are menopausal/post-menopausal?*

As you connect to the questions, or not, over the coming days, you may become aware of your dreams becoming more vivid, you may recall memories or feelings about your experiences.

I highly recommend that you keep your journal close at hand and note down anything that flows through.

You may also like to ask yourself:

- *What feels easy to me in this process?*
- *What am I resistant to?*
- *What feels difficult?*

Love and blessings to you, dear wise woman, I deeply honour your commitment to exploring these questions with me and allowing your voice to be heard.

I then contacted each woman to schedule a get-together, either online or in person where possible, for a conversation using the prompts, questions and their reflections.

Most of the conversations were in two parts and some with a year between each. This was not planned but was perfect in relation to the significance of how we change throughout our initiation.

I am profoundly grateful to the eleven women who shared their story with such integrity, candour, courage and joy. There were tears and laughter, rage and rapture, questions and answers as they revisited their menarche, menstruation, and explored what it is to be a changing woman.

Although each woman was asked the same questions and given the same prompts, there was not a rigidity to them. There was room to flow and freedom to wander as they spoke. Each interview began with a womb meditation.

Before you dive into the wisdom of the eleven women I interviewed, I felt it important to share my own story first. A wise woman sister suggested it may be more powerful to answer the questions in interview (rather than on my own), as each of the eleven women had done with me. This sounded like a perfect opportunity to be heard by a loving, listening heart. I know well the potency of allowing our voice to flow as we are being witnessed and heard by a tender sister. This is, after all, the work I do with women.

So, here first is my story, uncensored, authentic, light and dark, healed and healing.

BRIER

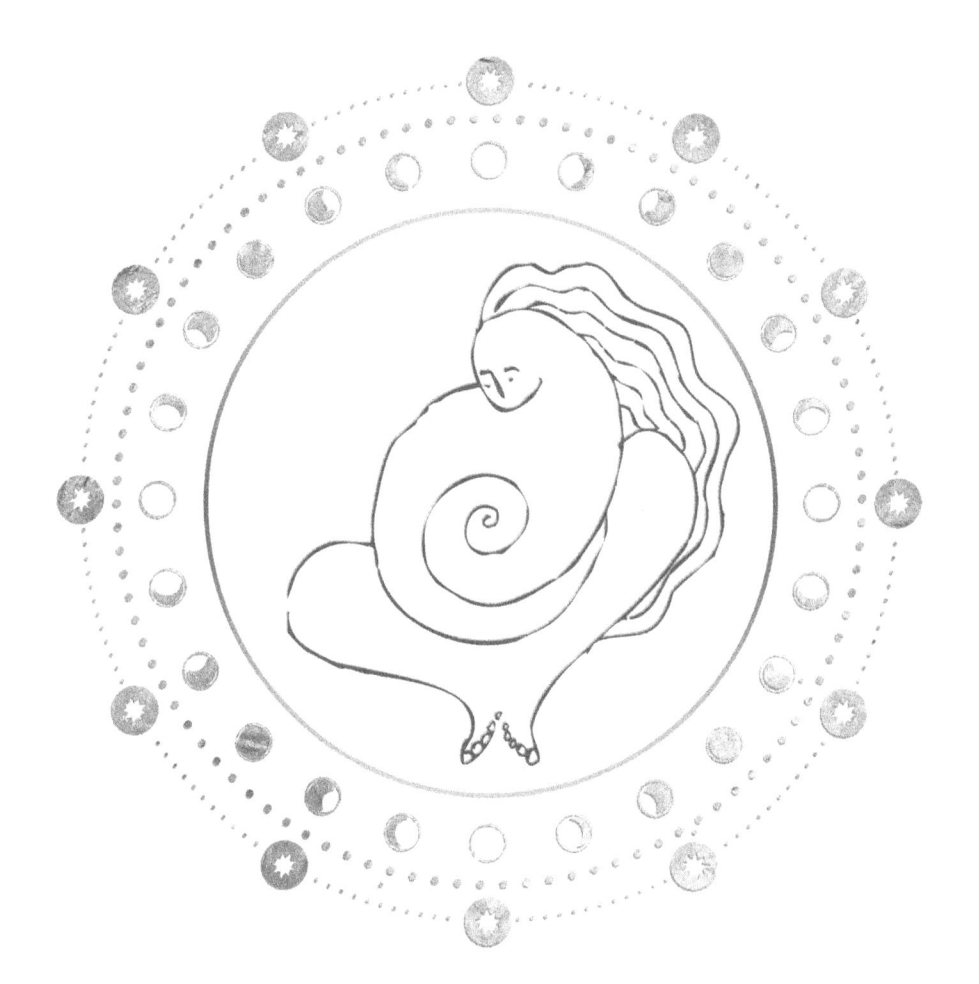

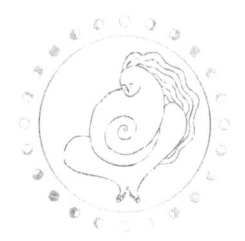

Wow, just doing that meditation with you Nicola, I can feel all eleven of you women, your voices, I'm tingling all over.

Oh, yeah, powerful, I can feel it too.

Okay, so Brier, what were you told, or taught, about what it is to be a woman, those first messages given by your mother, father, friends, media, society?

It's so huge this, isn't it? I've been giving a lot of thought to it.

I remember the innocence of being a child, just the sheer delight and magic of being a child. And actually summer, I was thinking about this sitting in the sunshine this morning, summer always signified, and still does, that sense of playfulness, of being a child. Summer is so abundant. I was very connected to that as a child. Some of that was innate, that innocence and still being attuned to my wild self, loving the softness of nature. I talked with the fairies and little creatures, I made up stories of adventures in foreign, distant lands. I enjoyed running through woodland, rubbing dirt in my face for camouflage, leaping over ditches like a warrior.

I want to honour my mum in that. She loved nature too and she modelled that to me. She spoke of the flowers and bird song; she spoke of the sky. So that was really beautiful.

But then, it changed as I grew up, the messages I was given. In my teenage years I had a strong urge to rebel against what I perceived as the bindings of being a young woman at that time, although I wasn't able to articulate it that way then.

I could feel my wild self being slowly eradicated.

I was expected to be feminine, a 'proper girl', which meant wearing dresses and being pretty. I remember going to a friend's birthday party which was being held outside in her garden. I asked my mum if I could have a new pair of corduroys for the party. I loved my brown corduroys.

But the mother of my friend admonished me, in front of everyone, for not wearing a pretty party dress. For not looking pretty. Clearly that comment went in at a very deep level, because I recall it.

The generation I was born into, I was born in 1961, it was still very much that the mother stayed at home and brought up the children. If she worked it was a part time job, to make a *little bit of spending money*. My mum worked for a while at the play group I went to. She also did the Tupperware parties and Avon Lady and Pippa D. Do you remember the Pippa D?

Yeah, I do.

She was a representative for all of those at various times, I don't think she did any of them for very long. But those were the types of things a mother was allowed to do because it didn't interfere too much with her being a mother and a wife. I find it so sad that being a mother, the primary carer and educator of our children was not valued for what it is, such an incredibly important and demanding role.

My dad's role, he got up early to commute to London (from Essex) and he got back late, after we had already had our baths and tea. He'd be tired and more often than not he'd be irritable. If there were toys on the floor he'd huff and puff and be pissed off that everything wasn't neat and tidy. So, there were tensions with the roles they both felt they had to live up to.

Then in my teenage years, I think it became more about friends, what they thought and what they did. We were all developing at different paces. I was one of the last to start bleeding. One of the last to have breasts, one of the last to have a boyfriend. It was all about how I felt, observing the other young women in my peer group. They all seemed to be more advanced in the way of the world – that's what it looked like to me anyway.

And then, through the media, the seventies were just crap for women. Weren't they?

Uh huh.

How we managed to find our way to being the women we are today is quite phenomenal. Because it was the *Carry On* girls, *The Bennie Hill*

Show. It was all tits and arse and being there for the pleasure of the gaze of the man. It makes my skin crawl now to think of that. We would sit as a family, mum, dad, me and my two brothers, laughing at all that sexist crap, because that's what we were taught to do.

Yes, yeah.

It's obscene. And Page Three, I don't know, they may still have that, I don't look at newspapers. But all of it was tits and arse and women were sex objects.

Or to be mothers.

It didn't always feel safe being female. I had to question whether or not to walk down an alleyway. Should I walk home alone in the dark? Would it be impolite not to acknowledge the questions or advances of a man I didn't know, who wanted my attention as I travelled into town on a bus?

I know now, that it was a time when I lost my connection to my magical world. I lost sight of the world in which I could be an adventurer, a world in which I could be free to express myself without shame or fear of being shut down or in danger.

I felt uncomfortable in the gaze of some men. I was afraid of what the looks suggested. I felt like there was always something that was wanted from me and I was supposed to give it without question.

So, none of that was positive!

It wasn't until I had left home, I was in London at drama school in my early twenties and suddenly my world started to broaden out.

Being a woman, in terms of that place, drama school, it was very competitive. There was some bitchiness. Some of the women behaved in the way that we had been taught to behave, to mistrust each other. To be what you wanted to be, meant you had to squish everyone else down around you, a very patriarchal type of energy. It felt very uncomfortable.

I met the sister of a close male friend I was at drama school with. She was older than me. About eight years older, I think. She came from a really strong, Labour, working class background and she was a Feminist. She was the first Feminist I'd met. She opened things up for me to begin to think in a different way. I began to question why I felt unsafe walking home in the dark or on my own. I began to notice and dislike the sexism and derogatory attitudes and behaviours towards women from some men. I felt an inner knowing stirring that somehow, I had been misinformed about what I could be as a woman.

She alerted me to Toxic Shock Syndrome, caused by bleached tampons; the dangers of taking the Pill. She introduced me to politics – she brought politics into my life. So, I think from that point, yes, I began to think differently. But it took a long time, a long, long time to begin to know the impact of all those years of being shown and told the patriarchal lies about what women are.

You've alluded to it there, what was the impact on you, of those messages you soaked up as you transitioned from girl to woman?

It was having the magic and the wanderlust of life and of being so connected to nature be dissipated. None of that had any place in how I was supposed to be anymore. I always thought that having a boyfriend would make me complete, that it was important. I thought I needed to have a boyfriend in order to be a worthy woman. And so, when I did eventually have my first serious relationship at the end of drama school, in our last year we got together and stayed together for a further three years. We were playing at making house. We were so unsuited. I look back at that and think, 'Wow, that was so powerful,' the message that I should be in a serious relationship. I placed myself in that situation, and I knew it wasn't what I wanted. But because that's what I had been shown, that's what we do as a woman. I hadn't been shown anything else, apart from my Feminist friend. So, I had no idea about what else I could do.

That was tied into work too, the jobs I was looking for. Although in some ways that was great, I've never been stuck in one route of work. Partly because I didn't know what I wanted to do. I loved drama school, but I didn't really want to be an actor. The jobs I've had and the work I now do has very much evolved as I have, over many years. For that, I'm very grateful. When I look back, I can see that in some ways I was empowered. I made my own choices about what I did, once I had freed myself from the relationship. I released myself from the notion that to be with that guy was what I ought to be doing. When I left that relationship, a work colleague said to me,

"You're like a bird set free from its cage."

Oh, my goodness. I resonate with that so much Brier. That idea of playing house, I had a lightbulb moment for myself, realising that's exactly what I did. When I finished University, I wondered why I felt so lost and so trapped. Yet on the surface it was what I wanted. So, thank you for that.

It is extraordinary isn't it, the power of those lessons?

Yeah, it's like sleepwalking into it all.

What are your memories of your first bleed?

It was a weekend, because my dad and two brothers were downstairs in the lounge watching TV. I could hear them and the TV. I went to the loo and saw blood on the toilet paper. I was very aware of them being downstairs. I must have gone and got my mum and she showed me the drawer where the Dr White sanitary towels were kept. They were those big, thick things that you put onto a belt. Dear god! So it was that, and my mum telling me I needed 'to be careful of boys now' and it was always referred to as 'The Curse' because that had been her experience.

There was absolutely nothing to say – 'Wow,' or 'Now things are going to change for you.' Nothing about noticing my cycle, how my emotions may fluctuate. Nothing about the magic and wonder of being cyclical, being a woman now. It was The Curse; it was inconvenient and I hated it. I was always pissed off when I bled. Having a period at school was awful. We were teased by the boys, having to have a note for PE, so everyone knew. Having to run round a hockey field with these big pads on.

I really just needed to be still and rest but I had no consciousness about that. No consciousness about the gnarlyness of how I felt leading up to menstruation. I knew it was called PMT (pre-menstrual tension) but what that actually meant and how I could help myself throughout the changes of my cycle, every month for years and years was never discussed, never modelled. All I knew was that I would have The Curse each month and be called a bitch when I was pre-menstrual and told to pull myself together if I got angry, not to be a nasty girl. I would be told to go to my room and think about my behaviour, seriously!

It wasn't until I stepped over the threshold into my initiation that I discovered the magic of being cyclical, just as it was beginning to fall away. It was only then that I began to honour it, my menstrual blood.

How did your experience of your first bleed impact on you as you entered into The Menopause? How did you begin to discover the magic of it?

Well, that took time as well. First off, I didn't know for a long time that I was perimenopausal. My periods were becoming heavy and painful, which I hadn't had for years, not since I first started bleeding. I knew there was something going on, but at that time my default was always to relate physical change to illness, that something was wrong with me. I phoned the NHS (National Health Service) Helpline one evening because I was afraid of the pain I was experiencing. The nurse suggested I go and see my GP, have a conversation, maybe a referral for a check-up. Which I didn't do. I wouldn't go there. I was too afraid. I was also at this time getting, oh my goodness, the rage. Oh my goddess, the rage I felt. Just wanting to rip people's heads off – well my husband's head off mostly. Because it was at that point, all the wounding was making itself known, which I didn't know. I didn't understand it as that then. He and I carried our own wounding in our relationship of course. We'd been together for a very long time.

So, what it was that changed everything, was having a uterine fibroid. When I got to Wales, I was already in the tornado. I brought myself here, to West Wales.

Which is interesting timing, that you'd made that transition to Wales as you were transitioning in Menopause.

Yes, absolutely. It was a calling. My innate wisdom, my intuition absolutely knew. My Wild Wise self, knew in my bones I needed to break away from where I was, and this is where I needed to be. An opening happened. I met women who guided me to the Circle I sat in for five years, which held me in a way that I was then able to find out what was going on, physically, mentally, soulfully. I then had the courage to go and have a check-up and was told I had a large uterine fibroid.

I immediately entered onto my healing pathways. I became a Moon Mother and learnt how to give and receive Womb Healings and Womb Blessings. I learnt to look at the stuff that I needed to look at. The wounding – it was time to heal the wounding.

For the first time in my life at the age of fifty-one, fifty-two, I began to love my menstrual cycle and my womb. Even though I'd had two children, who I grew in my womb, I still had never acknowledged my womb as the incredible creative force that it is, the power of my womb energy. Once I came to love my blood, even though my cycle was already really erratic, I didn't want to let go of it because I'd just started to honour it. I think that's why I actually didn't stop bleeding until I was fifty-seven.

Yeah, I hear that, to keep that connection, that relationship going. Amazing. What had been the messages you had received about The Menopause? You said going through your isolation phase, perimenopause, you weren't aware of what was happening. So, can you remember your mother's experiences, the messages you picked up?

My mum had a hysterectomy when she was relatively young and probably unnecessarily. As you know, I was offered a hysterectomy when I was told I had the uterine fibroid. There was no need for one at all but every time I went for a routine check-up scan, I was asked did I want a hysterectomy? That makes me so angry.

I have no idea if my mum had her womb or her womb *and* her ovaries removed. So, I don't know if she went into menopausal changes straight away, I don't know how that unfolded for my mum. It's not something that we ever talked about.

I remember her having rages. She was on anti-depressants for years, as so many women of her generation were. And menopausal women are still prescribed anti-depressants and hysterectomies. But we never talked about any of it.

I think there were things, maybe I do remember her having hot flushes and people laughing at it and being disrespectful of it, not from me. I think if anything came from me, it would have been annoyance toward her. We had that type of relationship at that time.

I don't recall any conversations between my mum and me or with her friends, never between me and my friends about The Menopause. It was nowhere on the radar.

Actually, I do remember when I was an older adult, talking to mum about hysterectomies. I was expressing how awful I found it that women were still offered them as a first option, even when the so called 'problem' was no danger to their health, and that there was no aftercare. She asked me what I meant. I said I meant that women were still having their wombs cut out unnecessarily and that there is no time or space given for the woman to grieve the loss of her womb, no support to heal from the emotional (and physical) wounding. She told me, "Well, we didn't make a fuss in my day."

I did once, try and open up a conversation with some very good friends, male and female, but the male in the group shut it down immediately. He said, 'I don't want to talk about the fucking Menopause.'

There must have been messages out in the media, in society, because all the women I've interviewed and myself included, we've all expressed that inner knowing that to be a menopausal woman we are going to be outwardly ridiculed and diminished. That's what we've learnt, even though it's not talked about. And we know that's not right.

It's so interesting, I'm meeting lots of women – they're coming to retreat at Spirals. They are all experiencing their disintegration. They have a session with me while they're here and a number of them hadn't realised until we started talking, that they are in their initiation, just as I hadn't, because in general, we are *still* not having the conversations that we need to have.

Had I not had my uterine fibroid; had I not come here, not sat in Circle with the women I did, not done the Moon Mother training and the other pieces I chose to do, I would not have understood my initiation in the way that I do, knowing it and experiencing it as the alchemical process that it is.

It is so interesting how we all picked up, like you say, those messages, but they weren't actually vocalised.

No and not under the label of The Menopause, I guess. But it was always very, very clear that as soon as we women started to lose our little girl peachy skin and our firm tits and to be the attractive female stereotype, we are no longer perceived as of any value as a woman. That message was so, so powerful throughout all of my life.

Yeah, yes, absolutely.

So, I think I know the answer to the next question! Are there aspects of The Menopause you enjoy?

I enjoyed thinking about this because in all honesty I've loved it all. Even in those moments, in that part of being in total disintegration and just not knowing myself. Obviously, in the moment it felt deeply uncomfortable and painful; there's grief and there's loss. But even within that, because I had chosen to be held throughout the unravelling, I knew that something magical was happening. I knew that this was my greatest healing. I knew that this was the gift of being given the opportunity to look at the wounding and really understand it and place it where it needed to now be. The image of a great oak tree is coming to mind as I say this.

Deep in my bones I knew I was healing and that always felt empowering. I loved how it brought me to sisterhood. Sharing my Menopause journey with other women was such beautiful medicine. This transformation also enabled me to heal my Mother Wounds, I came to understand how she had been silenced, how she had not been held, how she had not found spaciousness in which to heal her own wounding. I find that so very sad.

Finding my rage and being able to express it, at long last, was life changing. I shifted from a place of resentment, because I dared not speak my Truth, to being able to say, 'Fuck you,' to the patriarchal silencing. I felt the breaking of silence within my lineage. There was definitely some soul retrieval within that particular healing. Another step toward reclaiming my true nature.

The hot flushes, the insomnia, when I didn't know they were related to being a changing woman, I hated them. I thought, 'What's going on?' and 'I'm ill.' But when I knew what it was, I understood they were gifts and it was okay. I was able to regard insomnia as an invitation to meditate, to journal, to look at the night sky and gaze at the moon. And, I would think, 'Okay, if I can't sleep, what do I need to change during the day so that I'm not desperately exhausted and unable to function?' I know I was fortunate that at that point I had already chosen a life that allowed me to do that. I do realise that's not the case for every woman. Actually, for many women, as The Menopause comes in, they are at a point in their career where they're having to, or they are being told they have to, function in a very masculine energy. God forbid they have a hot flush, or sweat, or forget what the conversation is about in a meeting.

I think that has to change. Just as the attitudes toward menstruation have to change. It's long overdue that we give the respect our cyclical nature deserves. It ought never to be about a woman feeling she can't do her job anymore. It needs to be about attitudes and behaviours changing in the workplace, asking the question, how can we adapt the work place environment? How can we change things so that the value of who you are and what you know can still be within the work container? We need to ask, what can employers do differently to accommodate and support you in that, the changes women experience during their menopausal years?

So, yes, I loved it. I *still* get hot flushes. And I don't mind, I throw the covers off at night, I am curious about what the energy surge is bringing to me or telling me. I've learnt to listen to my body so much during my transformation. If I can't sleep, I'll write in my journal. I love that quiet time, on my own, to dream and to vision in those moments. Such magic comes in. I know I keep using the word magic, because it is. We are so in our potency and our power when we're menopausal and then when we become *Crone* – oh my goddess!

You know, I love life so much as a Crone woman; it's so beautiful. Whatever I feel, I *feel*, and it's okay because, of course, I still have moments where there are blips of doubt about whether or not I am capable, or worthy or good enough. But I understand it. There's a difference being in this place now so that when those things pop in, I can *be* with them and not freak out or fall apart as I did as a younger woman. I feel, what's the word? Is it 'agency'?

Yeah, that's a great word for it. That support and acceptance, when we're not accepting our experience, we can feel we're 'wrong' and look for ways to solve it and make it better. But that's where the alchemy is, in that acceptance, so powerful. You've said you loved it all. Was there anything, is there anything you dislike about The Menopause?

It's other people's responses to it I dislike. The fact that when I found out I had a uterine fibroid I was asked if I wanted a hysterectomy. My last bleed, I intuitively knew it was my last bleed, it went on for such a long time. I can't remember the exact time scale but for quite a chunk of time it was extremely heavy, and the bleeding just went on and on and on, I was exhausted. Intuitively I knew it was my last, but that voice of doubt, that powerful strong voice of, 'There's something wrong. You need to be checked out,' was very loud.

So, I had something called a hysteroscopy, which is a probe that is inserted into the cervix. I had this done twice. The first time the procedure was done by a woman consultant. She was lovely and the nurses were lovely. It was all pre-Covid. It was uncomfortable but it wasn't painful. And, everything was normal, my cervix, my womb, my ovaries. Then several years later I had some spotting. The medical profession says if you have spotting you should always have that checked out, by them.

Even though I'd already had the experience of my knowing the long bleed was my last and that I was healthy, again the, 'Oh there's spotting, there must be something wrong,' voice came in. And of course, as soon as you inform your doctor, they refer you to hospital for investigation. And you know, I didn't *have* to take the appointment, but I *did*. It was a male doctor this time, during Covid, so full protective clothing for them, masks for everyone. So, there I am, legs in the stirrups, so vulnerable, and he said, "I've done this xx amount of times and there's never been any problem."

Because there can be complications. In the literature they give you, it does say there are on occasions, problems which would require surgery.

He asked me if I'd taken any painkillers and I said, 'No.' I don't like putting pharmaceuticals in my body and the previous hysteroscopy hadn't been painful.

Oh, my dear. The pain. He couldn't get the fucking probe into my cervix. I had to rip my mask off. I had to find a way to survive that experience, actually. The way I did that was, connecting to myself at Soul level. I ripped the mask off and a guttural, primal sound was coming out. It was the sound of all of the women who have gone before me who have experienced abuse of their vaginas, their wombs, their cervix; and of abortion, difficult childbirth, whatever it may have been. It was all of that. It was my own knowing that I would not put myself in this situation again.

But I was there, and apart from shoving this man away from me, my only route through was to howl. Part of my brain was laughing because of what the consultant and nurses must have thought. I don't think they would have witnessed a shamanic releasing during the procedure before! The sound was from my Soul, from my womb, all the wounding of all women – that's what I experienced.

And, my cervix, womb and ovaries were fine, healthy.

Those procedures are the things I really disliked in response to my menopausal changes and the power of that voice. And I'm still working on that.

What is that voice?

The voice of the medical profession, the doctors. They are the perceived *authority* figures. That was what was taught to me. I'm not surprised I'm still having to work on that because it was what I grew up with. Not just from society as a whole but also within my family. My mother experienced illness for much of her life and she put such faith in the medical profession, external authorities, her doctors were God. I saw what that did to her over years and years of drugs and operations. It killed her prematurely, I have no doubt about that. I grew up with that model. That's what I witnessed, that was what I was taught. I had never been taught to trust my body, my intuition or my internal authority.

So, that voice is loud.

During lockdown, I experienced some discomfort in my left breast and immediately I went to my default of fear of illness. I have to say though, the voice was not as powerful on this occasion, not so dominant. I recognised it straight away as the 'voice,' and my intuitive voice is much clearer now. It's still a bit of a ping pong game.

Oh goodness. As you were describing that experience of the probe, I really felt like I needed to get up and move around, I could feel it in my body. It's like, the people in the room, the nurses, the consultant, they needed to have that experience, of that sound. Whether they knew what it was, who knows. But I wonder how that impacted on them and how much change they made.

Mmm, yes, I do wonder too. It's interesting that you say that because throughout the whole thing of having the uterine fibroid, I had to go back for regular scans, every three months to start with, then 6 months, then annually and then not at all. When I had the ultrasound scan, which was used to measure the size of the fibroid, I would speak to the nurses. I would say to them, "Everything is fine, there's no pain, no heavy bleeding," and that I put it down to the healing work I'd been doing.

"Oh. What's that then?" they'd ask.

"I've become a Moon Mother, so I'm working with the energy of my womb and the moon. And I sit in Circle with other women each month to dive into what needs to be looked at."

And I could see their faces glaze over with an expression of, 'What's she talking about?' They didn't know what to ask, so they asked nothing.

But I always felt that perhaps a little seed of curiosity had been planted. So, I do feel for each of the times I went and I spoke *my* Truth, of *my* experience that there may have been something for someone along the way which opened up a different enquiry.

That's so powerful. So, when you look in the mirror, what do you see?

I was going to be flippant and say that depends on whether it's a good hair day or a bad hair day! But there is some truth in that. I find this an interesting question, because now I feel much more at ease with how different I look. There's no denying, that when I look in the mirror, I am surprised not to see a younger me. Probably, I'd say around forty, between forty and fifty. Something that I've noticed, other women have said this to me, that with The Menopause, suddenly the aging process shows itself more quickly. Suddenly, I would look in the mirror in my mid to late fifties and think, 'Oh gosh, I don't look like I used to look at forty.' Of course I don't, because I'm an older woman.

Everything that I grew up with, that told us, when we start to lose our youthful looks became a nudge in my psyche. But it hasn't been such a huge thing for me in all honesty because I haven't believed in all that shit for a long time.

I see that I am an older woman. Increasingly, I enjoy seeing that and I enjoy that other people will see that I am an older woman too.

And, I see the life that I've lived in my face. I have a soft round belly now, which is fine, I'm stroking it now as I'm speaking to you. That's very different for me because I was always very slim and toned, that was my natural body. I never thought about what and how much I ate or drank; I always stayed the same size. It's different now.

I'm sixty and I know for my mother's generation, you were supposed to dress and look a certain way at this age. You were supposed to behave a certain way as an older woman. That is not on my radar at all. I love that I still wear exactly what I want to wear, how I want to wear it and where I want to wear it. I love not being bothered with make-up anymore, not that I ever wore lots of make-up, but I don't bother at all now.

I'm still waiting for my hair to go silver; I want my hair to be your gorgeous colour. It is slowly, slowly turning.

I see a wise, wild woman when I look in the mirror and I love her, I really love her.

Beautiful, that's what I see when I look at you as well.

Okay. So how do you feel about sex and sexuality as a post-menopausal woman?

It's interesting, because when I wrote *Take Off Your Armour*, I didn't speak about that. In the piece about The Menopause, I managed to skirt around it. But when it came to this book and I was putting the questions together to ask you wonderful women, I thought, 'It really has to be in there.' Because, like The Menopause, sex is something we don't talk about, not in my experience with my friends, and especially through our changing years. I think that's because having now talked with other women, we are expressing that our feelings towards sex really shift during our transition. Or they became more truthful, more honest actually.

So, for myself, I'm not interested in sex at all anymore. I'm just not. And I'm fine with that. It feels very powerful. I feel very clear about it emotionally and energetically, about what I want and what I don't want. But it's taken time to get there.

How I felt differently about sex was quite contentious between me and my husband for quite a few years, particularly during my isolation phase. It was difficult. Because it was tied into everything that was disintegrating, every aspect of our relationship was disintegrating. I think for him, it knocked him sideways, because at every level he is a physical person. It's who he is at Soul level, how he connects to the world. That's why he likes to build and to grow food and physical contact comes into that as well. So, it was very difficult. He felt it as a rejection of *him* when I expressed I did not want sex anymore. For a number of years, he just didn't understand. I got to the point when I felt if he didn't start to get this, our relationship wouldn't survive. He needed to do his own healing in relation to many things, his own disintegration if you like.

For me, I felt if he persists in challenging how I feel about it, not wanting sex, I'm done, because not he, not anybody was going to persuade me to feel differently about my body, my emotions, how I feel about sex now. This was *my* decision. Not anybody else's. So that was tricky. And we worked through it. When he eventually stepped over the threshold and onto his own pathway of healing his wounding, we came to a place of managing that particular aspect.

I know he still desires me physically and he would love the sexual part of our relationship to be there. And, you know, never say never! I don't know, who knows, but right now I have no interest at all.

It's interesting too, that when my sexual desire started to drop away, my own questions about myself came in. It was really fascinating. I thought, 'Oh, I don't want to have sex with the person I love.' I still loved him, I've always loved him. I can look at him and think he's gorgeous. But I don't want to have sex with him. Do I want to have sex with someone else? Do I want to have sex with a woman? Do I want to experiment and try some different things? Is that what it's about? Surely it can't just be, 'I don't want sex'? Because again, that's a message we're given, isn't it?

Yup, absolutely.

And actually, that's a piece that made me angry. Not only do we have the message within a patriarchal society, that as women we're supposed to be primarily sexual but also, within the wellbeing and spiritual community, I've heard some men, saying, 'Oh we can all enjoy a full sexual relationship up until the point we're going to die.'

When I hear that, I think, 'Hang on a second. How many conversations have you had with women? How many conversations have you had with menopausal women or post-menopausal women? Is this just your view that we should be wanting sex until we die?' And if we don't, then there's the view that something is wrong that needs fixing.

Yup. It's a huge thing that I've experienced in the spiritual community, and with women as well saying, 'Oh no, your sexual energy is your creative energy,' and, 'If you're not into sex then you're not open to everything.'

Even in relation to money we're told it's really important. You've got to have that sexual energy or it's a block.

Mmm, it's great that you've said that because actually, creatively, I feel *more* creatively open, a creative flow, than I have ever felt. I've always been a creative person but recently, changing my name, *that* unblocked something. It was very intentional as you know, and it's really opened up a flow of creativity and calling in those things that I want in my life. It feels really reciprocal, I'm calling it in because I want that and know I can be of benefit from what I give, what spirals out. And no sex involved in that at all!

Oh brilliant! Okay, so this may sound like a stupid question to you – do you feel connected to your womb energy?

Yeah, yeah, yeah! It's not a stupid question, because many of us don't. But yes, I do. Differently again. When I discovered I had the uterine fibroid I did the Moon Mother training and spent quite a number of years so focused on womb, for myself and healing for other women. The intensity – it's changed now – the intensity isn't there. It's much more, gentle. The connection is always there now. At first, I was having to learn it, I was having to re-wild. But now, the connection is there, that's not going away. What I find is, when there is a focus brought to the womb, such as when I'm doing a meditation with you in the Unbound community, it's 'boom,' the connection and focus is there immediately. And if I'm working with other women around womb, the connection and energy is just there, instantly.

And, I do still talk to my womb, I have my hands placed over my womb now, if I'm doing some dreaming or visioning work, I'll often start in my womb space. So, yeah, it's gentle, it's powerful and it's very beautiful. I love it.

I resonate with what you said there. When we first make that connection, there's a really passionate, intense relationship. And then it settles down. Then there's just that understanding there.

How about your yoni energy? Do you feel connected?

I do. I think that relates to what we've been talking about around sex. And, in relation to the hysteroscopies. It's an interesting one because when I was learning to reconnect to my womb, I didn't really look at my yoni energy. I guess the connection to my yoni has come more from those changes that I've just spoken about. I'd say I have less of a deep connection to my yoni than I do to my womb. It's still a piece that there's definitely space for looking at that really.

It's interesting answering this question because I'm realising there's been quite a lot of wounding around it. When I speak of the hysteroscopies, I can feel the wounding. My first child was born with ventouse and I was cut and had stitches. I tore giving birth to my daughter. I had an abortion in my early twenties. Years of having an annual Smear test. So, there's been a lot around my yoni energy that's been wounded. I certainly haven't looked at that in the same way as I had my womb wounding and healing. I'm glad you asked me that, I think that's something where there's space for exploration now.

So, final question. How do you feel now about being a woman, as a post-menopausal woman.

Well, so, so differently. From the point of menarche, to becoming a mother, to becoming menopausal, so different. I love being a woman. I don't want to paint a picture of me hating being a woman before becoming Crone. It really wasn't awful! I also enjoyed being a woman throughout all of that time as well, despite the shitty stuff.

But, to be a woman with the wisdom I have now is so different to being a woman with all of the repressive stuff we've been told, that shackled me in many ways, that's not my reality at all now.

My reality is, I love my feminine energy, I love my masculine energy; I've found a balance. It still shifts depending on what I'm doing, what I'm addressing, maybe who I'm with probably as well.

I have only recently realised that in all those years I was in full armour, fighting as an Inclusion Warrior, thinking I was standing firmly in my masculine energy – I wasn't at all. I was in the bath the other evening and had a download from which I finally understood I had been standing firmly in my feminine energy and what had been damaging to my wellbeing was that my feminine energy was battered by a predominantly masculine energy heavy world responding to my feminine energy. I was fighting linear, rational, analytical energy with compassionate, caring, nurturing energy. That's why I became burnt out. It was such a revelation to see this so clearly now all these years later.

I also feel a balance of the female archetypes. I have learned to call in and connect to each of them when I need to. I was missing my Maiden energy for so long, I love having her back, bringing in the playful, unbound flow and fantasy energy. I love the playfulness and the pleasure in just sitting and looking at a flower, feeling the sun on my face, the pleasure of getting my hands in the earth.

It's being able to embrace my Enchantress qualities, setting boundaries without having to be angry or diminish somebody else. I have learnt to set boundaries in a way that I know is right for me and I have the ability to be compassionate about it to support the other person to know that, that's my boundary!

And the Mothering, I love being a mother; and of course for me, I will always be called to my mother energy for my daughter. I love being a mother to my son. I love being a mother to other women.

I love sitting in my yurt with a woman I am working with and tuning in to her body language, having the ability to sense and feel her energy, intuiting what she knows, what she is yet to open to; all of those energies, I know are in myself too and are responding to her as I listen deeply, I just LOVE that, it's brilliant! I think, 'Yeah, there we go, at last!' The relief in not 'trying to be anybody' anymore. I'm not pushing, or thinking, 'Oh, can I do this?'

Now, I just show up and that's who I am.

I love being a post-menopausal woman, I love that I am in my Crone energy.

I love who I am and what I do. I feel such a profound connection to where I live, what I create, for myself, my family and the people who find their way to Spirals.

The experience of this initiation has been like no other in my life. Except perhaps the initiation of becoming a mother; being pregnant, in labour, giving birth and becoming a mother – that experience is comparable.

How powerful it would have been to have had that adventure being held in the way I was through my Menopause initiation.

Life excites me.

I am curious about what is yet to come, what my next initiation will be. Perhaps it will be death itself, leaving this body death, passing over.

I have been trying to find a single word to sum up how I feel post-menopausal, but there isn't just one. So, I think the following words sum up how I feel:-

Grounded, earthed, soulful, expansive, creative, joyful, spacious, alive, loving.

Beautiful. What a point to end on. That was amazing. Thankyou Brier, that was gorgeous. It gave me so much listening to you, so thank you again. So many lightbulbs going on! It's amazing how that happens.

Thank *you*. Yes, so many more conversations to be had.

Reflective Questions

What resonated with you from Brier's story?

What insights have you gleaned?

What is your biggest takeaway?

BEV

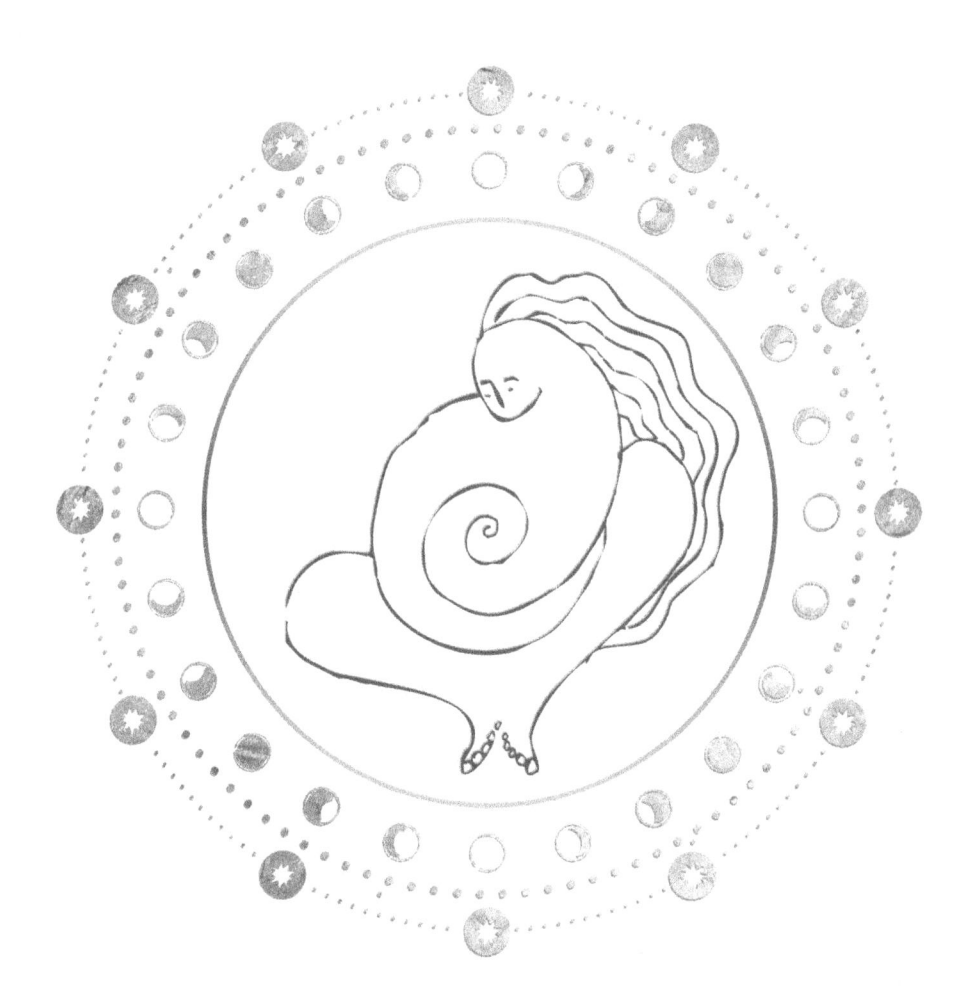

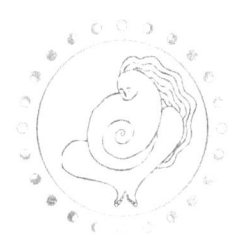

Welcome Bev, thank you so much for being here. I thought we would begin with the memory of your menarche, which you sent me some months ago. I was struck by how the question triggered such clarity in your memory and the excitement you felt as you relived that moment.

So, what do you remember about your menarche, your first bleed?

It's such a vivid memory, I remember so many details. The fact that I was wearing purple underwear, it wasn't obvious that it was blood that had made my underwear wet.

So, we were on a caravan holiday, I think in the Lake District. I don't think my sister was there. The normal routine was that we'd wake up, go to the shower block, get washed and dressed, come back and have breakfast. I'd gone off to the shower block on my own. I went to the toilet and I thought, 'Oh God, my pants are wet!' I thought, 'How embarrassing. I'm well past the age of bed wetting.' I had my shower, didn't notice anything else untoward while I was washing. I went back to the caravan, and again, I remember vividly, I had a sleeping bag, chocolate brown on the outside and yellow on the inside. So, I unzip it, throw it open to check the damage. And at that moment, my mum happened to notice, because that wasn't the normal routine. We'd usually just get on with the day, and mum probably had an instinct of what had happened and so she asked, "Are you alright darling?"

"Ah, no mum, I wet the bed."

She said, "Oh really?"

"Well, I thought I had but it seems okay."

And she said, "Look, I know this is awkward, but can I have a look?"

So, I said, "Alright then."

And she said, "Oh darling it's your period!"

I said, "Ohhh, right, okay!"

And literally with that, my dad walks in and says, "I'm going to the shops, does anybody want anything?"

And I answered, "Yes dad, can you get me some sanitary towels. I've just started my period and I haven't got anything." And mum's face fell and dad sort of embarrassedly cleared his throat and left.

Mum said, "Oh darling, you shouldn't have asked him that, he'll be really embarrassed. Don't worry, just use some tissues for now. We'll sort something when we go out."

I thought, 'Oh alright.'

In that moment, I didn't really think too much about it. I think possibly in later life I've looked back and thought, 'How sad.' Maybe when I was older and started going supermarket shopping, seeing men putting tampons into trolleys and thinking, 'Well, they're doing it now. Why couldn't my dad have done it then, you know?'

Back in those days we wore great big thick pads with hooks and elastic belts. I remember me and mum went out and had the whole shopping experience of getting that gear! And to be honest, that's about all I remember of my first blood. It's that initial awkwardness with my dad and it was never spoken of again. It wasn't a 'You mustn't talk about this.' We all took note that this wasn't something we spoke about together.

Something that did surprise me was, I went to an all-girl's school, and you would have thought, again with hindsight, we would all have been very open. But you would take your satchel to the toilet, you wouldn't just grab your Tampon or whatever and go, you'd take your whole satchel. So, it was obvious what you were doing but at the same time it wasn't obvious because we tried to hide it. And that surprises me when I think back. If it was a mixed school, fair enough, but we just didn't talk about it really. It wasn't till Mountview (drama school) that I started to talk to people about having periods and what it was like and stuff.

I was thinking about your story the other day and when you were describing how your dad walked in, for a moment I thought, 'Oh, yay, he's going to congratulate you and be happy to get your sanitary towels for you.' But of course he didn't, because he was of the generation that simply didn't talk about 'women's stuff.'

In the work I do, lots of women tell me how they felt shame about their menarche – the shame of bleeding. I wonder is that something you felt with your dad's response?

I didn't feel shame, it wasn't that. It was just something we didn't talk about. It was just factual. It was like we don't talk about the poo we did that morning. None of us felt the need to discuss it.

What surprised me when I started thinking through some of the other questions you gave me, was, in every other way, my dad was amazing. In terms of me being a woman, female, I was never treated like the second-class citizen, that maybe my mum's generation was, and it was probably because my dad had two daughters. I was encouraged to help him with all the DIY (do it yourself). I used to be the scraper, the sander – not so much about tinkering around with cars, but, yeah, I was sawing, I was drilling. I was like his little apprentice! So, in every other way he involved me and treated me like an equal. It was just that one little thing really, that made a difference. Which is a shame.

Did he involve you with these things before you started menstruating?

Yes.

So, he was already modelling to you that yes you were a girl but that didn't stand in his way or your way in doing things together that interested him and that you enjoyed. I wonder if that's the reason you didn't feel shame, because you had that solid relationship with your father where he included and valued you?

Possibly, yeah. I'm sure if he'd have had a son, I suspect we would have had a very different relationship. My older sister had a much more fractious relationship, being the eldest, she was the one pushing the boundaries. I was the one just toddling along, being the good girl, the baby sister, not causing any waves in the family.

Let's pick up on that 'good girl' piece then of how for our generation and even more so for our mother's generation, girls were meant to be 'sugar and spice and all things nice.' How much do you think you felt that, at the time and also in retrospect?

In retrospect, a lot. At the time, when I was very young, not. When I became a young teenager and in my mid-teens I was very good at playing the game of being a good girl, telling them what they wanted to hear. But I wasn't, I was taking drugs. I was having sex but as far as my parents were concerned, they thought I didn't drink or do any of what I was doing! So, I was very aware of playing the role of the good girl.

With hindsight, I am aware I flirted with my dad, I've read lots of girls, daughters, practice their flirting skills on their dad. I'm aware I did that. I remember saying things to him like, 'I wish I could marry you when I grow up' and him having to explain to me why that wouldn't be possible and me not really getting it at the time. I probably was a bit of a daddy's girl, but I was also very close to my mum. Which I suppose is a bit unusual.

Did you have conversations with your mum about your blood as you grew up, your sexuality or your boyfriends as you were growing up?

No. My sister had a drive to be totally honest and tell them everything and I saw all the problems that created, to the point that mum was taking Valium. She was of that generation when if you said you can't cope, you're given tranquillisers. So, the message I got was, 'Don't tell them, it just creates too many problems.'

I talked a lot to my sister. I have a vivid memory of being in the bathroom with her. She was explaining to me what the lyrics of David Bowie's song, 'Aladdin Sane,' meant, you know, 'Boys wanking to the floor,' 'She comes, she goes.' She explained all the sexual lyrics in detail! Most of my sexual education came from my sister. We had very open conversations about it. Not about being straight, or gay or bi, I just didn't have that type of awareness, not until I got to drama school. Up to then the only thing I saw were 'camp' entertainers on TV. Drama school was a real eye-opener.

So, thinking about how you didn't discuss any of this with your parents because it didn't feel safe to do so, how do you think their messages and behaviours impacted on you? How did you perceive yourself as a young woman as you arrived at drama school, your first time living away from home?

I was very sexual, pre-Mountview and at Mountview. You ask a question towards the end of your prompts about sexuality as a menopausal woman – and to be honest I don't really feel I have a sex life, but not in a negative way. It's sort of like, I'm done with it, but it's not like, 'Oh I want it and I can't have it.' It's, 'Yeah, been there, done that.'

It made me think back to *why* I was so sexual as a young woman, and I think it was partly the times, because we could. We had the Pill, it was pre-AIDS (Acquired Immune Deficiency Syndrome). It was like, why bother restraining yourself? – If you feel the urge, go for it. But it was also about, for me, I loved being held, being accepted. That for me I think was *more* of what it was about. It was about people showing a form of acceptance for me.

Now where that comes from, I'm not totally sure.

Dad was ex-military. He had a very strict Victorian upbringing. Military was who he was. He was very stiff upper lip, we're British, keep it all buttoned in. But all hell let loose in the Officers Mess! I remember him telling me all sorts of stories of the fun and games they got up to there, but we never saw that side of him. That was very much what he did with the boys, not as a family man.

Mum had a strict upbringing too. She was brought up during the War – Bristol Blitz. Her brother was killed by a bomb in the Blitz. Her mother turned round and said, "I wish it had been you." Which must have been heartbreaking. So, she spent her life seeking approval, because she didn't get it from her mother. She always kowtowed to dad because she couldn't risk upsetting the applecart or not being the wife he wanted – so there was very much a sense of control in the family home.

The sexual thing was I think, me being a total rebel against everything mum and dad stood for, which was the *control*, doing things *properly*, being the *good girl*. I mean we weren't a religious family but we might as well have been. You know, no sex before marriage. I do remember when I did eventually tell them about Shane (a boyfriend from my early 20s), when we notionally got engaged and mum asking me, "Well, if you're engaged, does that mean you have relations?" or whatever words she chose to use.

And I said, "Well, yeah, actually we have." I thought, 'I'm 21 now, or near enough, I don't have to lie.'

I remember her saying, "You gave him your most precious possession."

I felt, 'Whoa, come on mum,' but that was her view of it.

So, the sexual stuff was about rebelling against my parents. And a bit came from my sister, because she did the whole thing of doing things properly and just got a load of stick for it anyway and she ended up leaving home under very unhappy circumstances. She practically ran away. She went off with her boyfriend. She timed it when mum and dad were at work. I was the only one there – I knew she'd gone. Mum and dad didn't know she was going. It was all very acrimonious and unpleasant. I think some of that was payback to mum and dad. My sister did the right thing and look how they treated her. They thought I was wonderful, but actually I was doing worse things than she was doing. It was all a bit convoluted really.

But, being a grown up now, I don't need any of that. I don't play games anymore. I don't need to seek approval. I really am comfortable with who I am, I feel, as a post-menopausal woman, amazing and wonderful and sort of wish I had got to this point years ago. I don't give a fuck what anybody thinks of me anymore.

And that is the beauty of becoming Crone.

And they don't tell you about it!

What I knew about The Menopause, was all the medical stuff, the physical stuff – the foggy memory, hot flushes, the aches, the mood swings, the hormonal kick off. No-one ever told me I was going to feel *amazing* once I got through to the other side, and that I'd feel more confident than I've ever felt in my life before, emotionally stronger than I've ever felt in my life before, I love it.

I felt a little bit uncomfortable getting to this point, because of the physical stuff, you know. I did play around with HRT for a little bit, with diet and exercise and stuff. A combination of the passage of time and various things and I've come out the other side, and it's like, 'Whoa, this is amazing.' I love it.

I think the other benefit of being an older woman, and maybe I feel this more being in London, you become invisible. Nobody sees me if I'm on the Tube or walking down Oxford St. Nobody sees me, nobody's clocking me, not like when I was a young woman. When you're a young woman, men are checking you out, 'What does she look like? Is she fit? Do I fancy her?' Other women are checking you out, 'Is she a threat to me? Is she better looking than me?' Whereas now, I feel people just don't notice me, which is lovely, because I can just slip into the shadow and I can observe, especially when I go out and do photography. I can just stand in the background – people just do not see me. I get some lovely photos and stuff, and I actually like that. There was a little moment when I thought I'm not sure if I like this or not, but now I do. I do actually like not being noticed anymore, just being part of the crowd that no-one's really aware of.

That's so interesting to hear you say that, because I think many women do feel they become invisible. Because society has been shown and told that elder women are not attractive, or desirable or sexual or sensuous and that we're crazy; all of those really negative messages, whether we are consciously aware of that or not. It's all there in what we've been told and taught. And I think that impacts on how we experience our menopausal years. I have to say, I don't feel invisible, I do feel men look at me differently and what I like about that is that they have an opportunity to see the wise Crone woman, who is still sensual and is still attractive.

I'm talking more about the people I *don't know*, people on the Tube, people I pass on the street. Within my circle of friends, it's different sometimes. At a gathering there was a guy I run with. He got very drunk and he was flirting with me and told me how sexy I am, so within my immediate circle of friends, I don't feel invisible with *them*, just out in the wider world.

So, let's look at your relationship with your womb and yoni. Do you feel you have one?

I wouldn't say I *don't* have a relationship at all. Through my teens I had horrendously bad periods, to the point I was passing out at school, in absolute agony, bleeding very heavily. And eventually I was put on the Pill (I was 15), which was the beginning of all the sexuality. That was the only way my GP said it would be sorted and the benefit of that, was the conversation was said in front of my mum! So, my mum knew I was on the Pill, I didn't have to hide it or pretend or anything. Perfect timing from a sexual point of view.

For a lot of the time, I used to take the Pill continuously, so I wouldn't have a period, because they were just devastating for me. I hated having them. That carried on pretty much until I met Alan, my husband, aged 23. And because I was with someone who loved and cherished me and someone

I felt safe with, I carried on taking the Pill, just as a contraceptive, because I didn't want to get pregnant. And I think I did start having periods more normally and actually realised they weren't so bad. I don't know if it was because I was older or because I was taking the Pill or whatever.

So, my mid years I had my daughter Lucy and from a womb point of view it was, 'My God, you're amazing, look what you've done!' I probably didn't acknowledge that at the time, but with hindsight, that is such an amazing thing. You have two people, then you have three! *My* body made that happen. Okay, Alan needed to do his little bit, but my womb grew this human being, who is the light of my life in every respect. So, yes, I have amazing respect for my womb because of that.

With the onset of perimenopause, I went back to the teens again with horrifically painful periods, very heavy bleeding. I had one horrendous incident, when I went to meet a friend at Pizza Express after work. When I got there, I went to the bathroom to change my pad, I had stopped using tampons a long time ago. I had an overnight heavy-duty pad on. We had our meal over an hour and half maybe, and as I stood up at the end of the meal, I had soaked through everything, covered the chair. I was mortified, but luckily, an angel came – otherwise known as a waitress – and I said to her, "I am so sorry, could you get me a damp cloth. I need to clean this seat."

And she said nothing, she smiled, she went away. Came back with a cloth. She moved to do it. I said, "No, no, let me clean that, thank you."

I happened to go back there a month later and got the same waitress. I don't think she remembered me, but I left her a massive tip and she said, "Really?"

I said, "Yes, you were so kind to me last time I was here."

I don't think in that moment she remembered or it wasn't a big deal for her. It was a *major* deal for me. The only benefit for that day was I was wearing black trousers, rather than a yellow skirt or something, but I remember I grabbed a free newspaper on the Tube and put that on the seat and sat on it on the way home, all the way home, I was embarrassed. Maybe I shouldn't have been, it's a perfectly natural thing, but I was.

As my periods were coming to an end and all the hormonal stuff was kicking in, the first symptom I had, at the beginning, was night sweats. Not so much the hot flushes in the day. It was the night sweats, when I'd literally wake up on fire, soaked. I don't think I had a decent night's sleep for months. I'm not good with lack of sleep. I start to fall apart. And that's when I went to the doctor and said, "Look, I need some help here!"

I wasn't sure about HRT. When I stopped taking the Pill, I didn't go back on the Pill after having Lucy. We used condoms and calendars and stuff. I had got to a point when I didn't like putting drugs in me, unless it was necessary.

So, I was very much in two minds about HRT. But I was also a little bit desperate. I need to sleep. I can't function without sleep. My doctor was really good. She talked me through all the pros and cons, like the risk of breast cancer and everything, and I said, "Well look, can I try it for a while and then come off it and see how I go?"

I think I was on HRT for about nine months, which sort of got me back on an even keel, and then I gradually reduced the dose to one every other day, half every other day and then three days between them and gradually weened myself off it. I think I only took it for about nine months, and that was just enough to get me over the worst. I do still have the very occasional symptom but they are literally like once or twice a week, I just love being the other side of it really.

When you went to your doctor, was HRT the only thing she offered you?

No, that was when my health and fitness thing kicked off around 2015. She just made this passing comment. She didn't make a big deal out of it, she just said, "If you lost a few pounds that might help."

And that was all she said, she didn't make a big deal out of it. I went away, and you know when someone makes a comment and you replay it later? I looked in the mirror and I thought, 'Yeah, you are a bit chunky Bev. It wouldn't do you any harm.' So, I started eating sensibly, that's when the running started and I lost weight and I think that definitely helped as well as the HRT. I think it was the combination. When I came off the HRT, I was slimmer, I was healthier, I was eating better. I think it all just came together. She didn't *sell* HRT to me. For me it was, 'I'm desperate, I need this sorted, I can't function at work, I'm tearful,' and it was all down to not sleeping. I needed to sleep, but I didn't want to take sleeping tablets. For my mind,

HRT was the lesser of two evils.

But yes, she was good, she did talk me through all the various options. She did also say Black Cohosh, Red Clover may help and talked about those as well. I have taken those on and off when I finished HRT and things weren't quite running as smoothly. I still take to this day something called Menopace, which is a bit of a combination supplement. Again, I tried to come off it last year, I did a similar thing just cutting down the dose and leaving more and more days between and then after a while I was feeling lethargic. I was feeling miserable and I thought, 'Where's this come from?' And I thought, 'Oh I wonder, I've stopped taking Menopace,' and I started taking it more regularly again. I felt better and I thought I'll take this for a while and see how we go.

There's a really good book if you're interested called 'Menopause Years: The Wise Woman Way,' by Susun S Weed. I dip in and out of it to support me through various stages and phases. First of all, she looks at herbal remedies and then supplements and then the doctors, GPs, HRT. I found it really useful.

Mmm, yeah, I'd be interested in that.

I want to pick up on what you said about insomnia. So many women who are going through The Menopause experience insomnia. I had dreadful insomnia, and I didn't realise I was menopausal because I had very regular bleeding up until I was 57. I really fought against it for a long, long time and then when I started to do the work that I do, I got into trying practices like journaling and recording my dreams. I always have a note book by my bed now. Or sometimes it was just sitting up and opening my curtains to look at the night sky.

Did you rest during your changes? I'm really interested to hear from you as a woman who works in the corporate sector; having to look a certain way I assume, having to work regular hours, probably long hours, holding meetings. Having to have a particular persona perhaps for the work that you do. I'm really interested to know, how did you manage that, or how are you managing that?

Well, that was part of the reason why I had to go on the HRT, because I wasn't functioning due to the lack of sleep. But night sweats were *always* the worst thing. So, during the day I was okay, and I've not really had the hot flush thing, I get it occasionally, but during the day I was fine. The bleeding, I think because I've always had heavy periods, I was sort of okay with too. Because I'm office based, it was quite easy to nip in and out of the bathroom to do what I needed to do and luckily, we had a bathroom where there was a sink in with the toilet. So that wasn't such a big deal for me. We even had a little medicine cupboard in the bathroom to keep my supplies in, so there was no walking to the toilet and everyone knowing what you were doing.

But also, I think because with me and The Menopause – becoming more confident was actually part of that journey. It also helped that my Senior Director (male) is about two years older than me, and we have a very friendly relationship, so I never felt my age was a problem. I never felt being an older woman is a problem there. Other companies yes, but not where I am now.

So, I'm quite comfortable making a joke, saying things like, "Oh, ignore me I'm just an old woman, I don't know what I'm talking about," or "Ignore me, I'm having a hot flush."

I don't have a problem with that side of things, not in this job, because I don't feel like I'm going to be judged for it. In fact, they were very supportive when I said I wanted to start running and when that led into coaching, because that became a second job, and so, (because of their) Terms and Conditions, I had to get their approval. I said, "I've been invited to be a Running Coach. I'd love to do it, but it will mean I'll have to leave early on a Thursday, how do you feel about that?"

And they were fine. My boss is a Gym Bunny. He's at the gym every morning and he said, "Bev, if it's to do with your health and fitness, I support you all the way."

They've always been very supportive and encouraging. I'm lucky in lots of ways with this job. I couldn't do it if I hadn't done all the other things I experienced in my earlier years. It's a job where being a Crone is an advantage. Because it's about having experience of work and life. Operations Manager is the role I have. It's about sorting things out, when things go wrong. I'm treated like the mother in the office. It's like, 'Bev will sort it,' 'Bev knows what to do,' 'We can count on Bev.'

When I go on holiday, it's like the mother leaving the nest for a little while. But it's the perfect job for me at this age. It plays to all my strengths. It only challenges me in terms of learning new ways of doing something I've done before or learning new language around the products. But that helps build my confidence as well.

I love that you put the word Mother into the Menopause piece because I feel very strongly that when we are Crone, we are the Mother of the World, Mother of Earth bringing our wisdom out into the world in order to hold others and to gift to them our wisdom, our experience and that's such a beautiful thing that we bring to the world.

Whereas perimenopause is the disintegration of self. To begin with, because I didn't really know what was going on, that was incredibly difficult. I'm interested to know; did you experience any of that?

Not as consciously and not as overtly. I think my transition happened, and I don't know that it was specifically Menopause, when I started running. When I was at Mountview, I danced quite a lot there but after that, I did zero exercise until I started running a few years ago. So, it was a whole new thing and not something I thought I was ever cut out for. But doing the course, that I now coach, I was taught *how* to run.

And that's where my transition has come from because I love running on my own. I find it hypnotic, I find it meditative because my body falls into this rhythm and I'm doing it over and over again, one foot in front of the other, one foot in front of the other, so my body's busy. My body knows what it has to do, it gets on with it. And this allows my brain to wander, to go off wherever it wants to go. And in fact, this is where my tension, if I can't run for a while, that's where my tension comes in and it's not so much that I haven't done the *physical* thing of running. It's because I haven't done the *mental* thing of running.

And I don't necessarily set out with a question to answer or a problem to solve. I just go out and as I'm running, life gets better, one way or another. I described it to somebody as water going through a filter. Do you remember the filter beds in geography lessons at school, where you've got the big stones and then smaller stones and then tiny stones and then the sand? And the water starts at the top and goes out at the bottom. As it flows through, it leaves behind all the sludge. And that's sort of what happens to me when I'm running. So, whatever is in my head, goes down through these filters, and the thing is still there, the thing is still real, but it's not such a big deal anymore.

Earlier this year I got really close, closest to being depressed than I have for a while. Last year we had a lot of building work done at home, there was a whole lot of stuff going on. It took the best part of a year. It was also Lucy's wedding, so there was tons of stuff going on last year. Alan was diagnosed as having COPD (Chronic obstructive pulmonary disease).

So, at the beginning of this year, I was sort of at a loose end, I didn't have a project anymore, there wasn't a wedding, the house was done. My mind just started to play on, 'Well, dad's 90, mum's 89, they're not going to be here too much longer. My cat Tilly is 15. She's not going to be here too much longer.' And then I did the stupid thing of Googling Alan's condition and seeing that typically it's a five-year prognosis. It could be less if someone's not in good health, which he isn't. And I thought, 'Oh, great, that's what my life holds now – just saying goodbye to too many people I'm close to and my cat.' And I got really, really down and depressed. But one of the things that got me through it was running. I would go out and would just run. And that built up my mental strength again. Distance running is where my mental health comes from. It is definitely *my* spiritual thing.

So, perimenopause, I didn't fall apart in that way. For me it was mainly physical, the very heavy periods, the hot flushes, the sweats at night, not being able to sleep. But the more mental transition comes from the running side of things.

How old were you when you identified for yourself that you were menopausal?

A couple of years before I started running, so about 2013. So, I would have been 52, 53. And I haven't had a bleed for about three years now. When I came off HRT it just stopped, there were no more.

Well, here we are at the last question. When you look in the mirror what do you see?

Do you know this was the hardest question for me to answer and I just put 'me'! I'm not sure what else to say.

I'm happy with who I am. I'm happy with what I look like now. I haven't been in the past, when I was very overweight. But I see strength from the muscles in my legs from running.

Yeah, I'd like not to have a saggy neck and all the wrinkles but, that's who

I am, part of who I am and I like who I am. So, I take the good with the bad really. I think that's where I am with how I look.

Thank you so much Bev. It has been so interesting to hear how you have travelled through your changes. Your running practice sounds so incredibly powerful, I am sure what you have described will be wonderful medicine for other women.

Reflective Questions

What resonated with you from Bev's story?

What insights have you gleaned?

What is your biggest takeaway?

JENNY

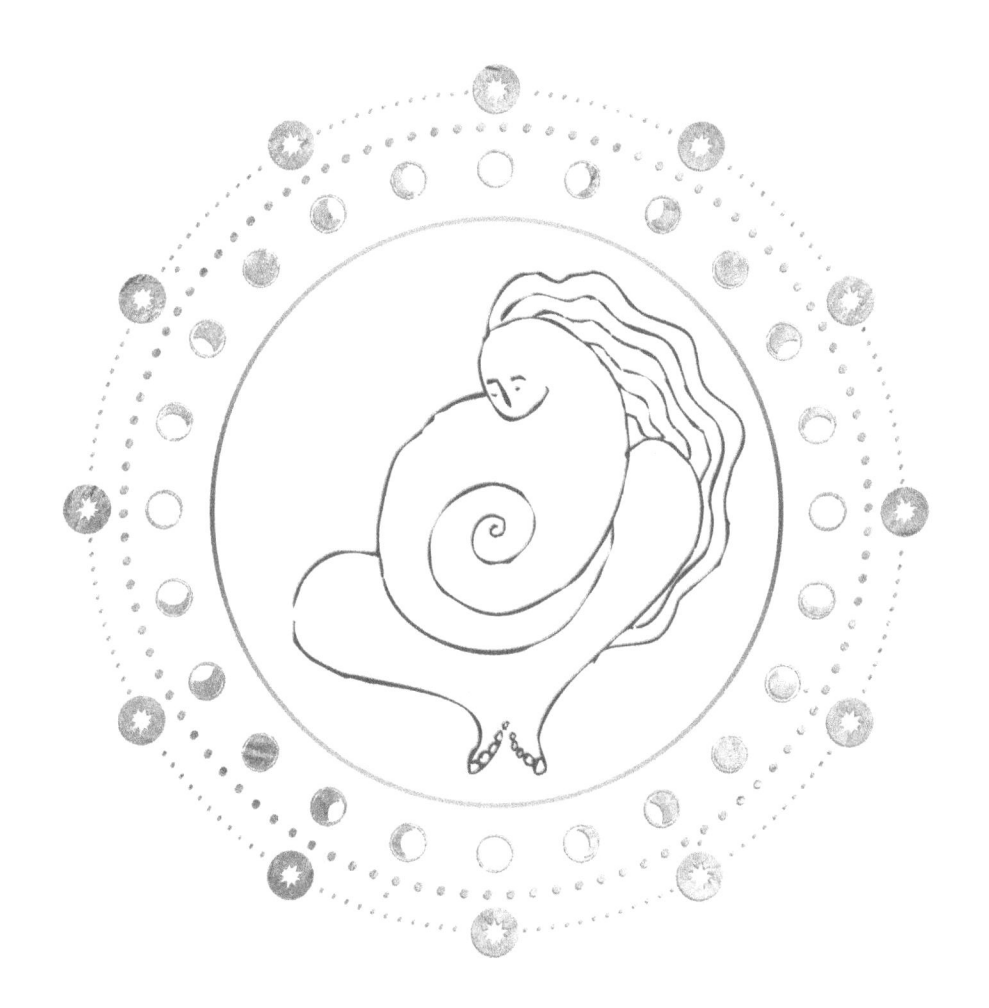

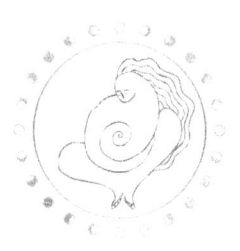

What have you been told or taught about what it is to be a woman – through the media, parents, friends?

I really don't remember anything from the media. Looking back, I don't think I saw anything on TV or listened to anything that felt relevant. So, it was more about what I picked up from my mum and friends really. From my mum a feeling I got, through her showing and expressing things was, 'You just get on with it.'

With being a woman?

With being a woman, yes. A big part I picked up on was nurturing and looking after others.

In the sense of that's what she did or that's a woman's responsibility?

Both. I picked up that's what she did. It impressed upon me; it was very much about nutritionally looking after the family, making sure they were provided for, nurturing from a more physical way, rather than emotional, I suppose. Being a woman from her generation, my mum gave up work when she married. She never worked throughout the whole of my parent's marriage. She was very fastidious about her looks and looking pretty and having a very clean house. That was more important to her than looking after our emotional needs, me and my sister.

Did she do those things with joy, or was it with resentment – maybe something in between?

It was a mix. Some of it felt like she was on automatic pilot. But she loved cooking; she became a good cook. She enjoyed cooking – we weren't allowed to get in her way – she did it on her own. For me, I picked up 'duty' from her. A duty to get the housework done. So, that was done like a duty, being on automatic pilot, doing what her mother had been and done.

I felt, womanhood was about finding love, connecting with a man, perhaps. It was more about finding another connection. It was about getting attention at that time. It was less about the sexual feelings and more about getting attention.

Was this as a girl or as a woman?

As I was transforming really – as an older teenager. I had quite a lonely childhood really. My sister and I are seven years apart, and we lived right in the middle of nowhere, so I had to rely on my parents to give me lifts to places. I spent a lot of time on my own. I was quite withdrawn, I suppose, from my parents. Spending more time with my friends, was an opportunity for more independence, as I was getting older. Which wasn't easy because we lived in the middle of nowhere. So, I realised then I was really craving attention, because I wasn't getting it from my mum.

I'm wondering, you say that for your mum, her appearance and the state of the house was important to her, that it was a sense of duty and as you say, for our mother's generation that was very much seen as their role. So, how did that role model impact on you? Was there a time in your life when you looked at that and thought, 'That's for me,' or 'I really don't want that'? When did that happen for you, if it did?

Yeah, definitely, it did! For me it was definitely, 'I don't want that!' I think it was very slow. I don't remember ever thinking the other way. My sense was, I didn't want to be dependent, be like my mother, not working, dependent on a husband or a partner financially or otherwise. I got a feeling of, a sense of, if I became a 'housewife' like that, I'd feel trapped. Trapped at home, no connection with the outside.

And do you think that's what it was for your mother?

Well, when I was a young adult, we had a talk about motherhood and she admitted that she'd never wanted to be a mother. It's just what you did. And she said, "I wouldn't be without you both but that's just what you did."

So, there must have been some underlying, unspoken sense of what I was picking up.

How did that impact on you? In relation to your own feelings about being a woman?

To be a woman, to allow myself to follow that role of my mother, felt like we were a weaker sex, a dependent, trapped woman.

And so, did you think that's what women are? Did you think we are a weaker sex? Or were you thinking we are treated as a weaker sex?

No, I felt that her generation were treated as a weaker sex. I didn't feel that we were. And I felt that I had a choice and I chose not wanting to be a young mother, not being dependent on anyone. Not repeating the same process that my mother went into just because it was expected.

And what about your father? What sort of impression did he give you about what it is to be a woman?

I haven't really thought about it. I think the sense that I got from him was still to do with service, looking after the family. When I got to the point where I had to decide what career I wanted to do, he pushed me towards secretarial work because even though I didn't want to do it, it was a good profession to be in and something to fall back on. But that would have been being in service too, more than likely to a male boss. And all I wanted to do was travel, be a hotel receptionist or something in the travel industry, at that time.

When your dad got home from work was his expectation that the house would be clean and tidy and there'd be a meal on the table for him?

There was never any fall out about it. Mum got on with her job and that was her business. I don't ever remember my dad laying down the law about what needed to be done. She was the boss of her house; he was in charge of the garden. So, he was quite easy going like that. I don't ever remember him demanding food at a certain time.

How do you think these messages impacted on you as you transitioned from girl to woman? You've started to talk about recognising that their model was not what you wanted. Were there any messages that you saw or heard that showed you a different way a woman could be in the world? Or did this come from you instinctually, a part of your nature?

I think it was a rebellion thing going on inside. I had a year in boarding school when I was ten, which was a terrible time in my life. I felt extremely lonely, a very difficult time. I had to look after myself. I had to rely on *me*. There wasn't anyone else there as an emotional support at all. The resentment I felt when I was back in the family group again, and my parents were being quite strict with me. There was a sense of feeling trapped, not only from seeing my mother's perspective but from my own perspective of, 'Who are you to boss me about when I've had to fend for myself for a year?' There was this real fight to not be dominated, I suppose. Not being told what I needed to do was very strong in me.

My transition from girl to woman, I noticed that particularly being around my friends, particularly my best friend, I became more self-conscious about my looks. I became more creative with dressing up. I really loved drawing pictures of models and putting clothes on them, that was a very creative period for me. I was about fifteen years old. It would have been nice to follow up and be a fashion designer or something like that, but that wasn't thought of at the time. It was just a hobby I had.

Do you think that was about creating an expression of yourself? Who am I? How will I express who I am through my clothes? How I look?

Yeah, because I had moved around quite a lot, different schools, constantly changing friends. I realised I had my own ideas about how I wanted to look, how I wanted to dress and not to be a follower of fashion at all. That increased as I became more self-conscious and wanting to look nice and experiment with how I looked, my hair, my clothes. I really enjoyed learning about make-up and doing my own hair, finding my own creativity with it.

So, it was about you using that as a form of self-expression rather than, 'I'm supposed to be wearing make-up. I'm supposed to look a certain way'?

Yeah, definitely. It was my own wish. I wasn't a follower of any set way; I think I rebelled against the whole thing. Apart from enjoying being feminine, I suppose I was just more self-conscious of how I looked as I became a woman.

I enjoyed that time in my life because as I was starting to go out with boys, it gave me more independence really. The group of friends I had, some of them had their own cars, so it meant I could go out without my parents picking me up. I had more freedom.

When you started to go out with boys, what was that experience like for you? Did you have any expectations? Did the boy's you dated have any expectations? Can you say how that was for you?

I was taken by surprise actually by the sexual advances so quickly. I was really quite innocent and not knowing what to expect. My first boyfriend took me by surprise. I wasn't quite ready, not that he did a great deal, but I just couldn't find the words to say, 'No I'm not ready.' I was quite shy. It wasn't scary as such; I didn't get scared. It took me a little while to find my voice and my boundaries. I didn't have any bad experiences. It made me realise I needed to set my own boundaries.

Let's talk about your first bleed, do you remember how old you were?

I think I was fifteen.

So, that was about the same time that you started to express yourself through clothes and make-up and going out with boys. Can you recall the first time you menstruated, what that felt like, your mother's response to it? Did your father know? What were the attitudes of your friends like?

I remember I was at school. I was ill the day before I started menstruating, I thought I had some sort of bug. I got a temperature, I felt nauseous, I had a lot of pain down in my abdomen, back pain especially. I didn't quite know what was going on, I just felt rough. It was the next day at school that I suddenly started to bleed. I didn't have anything with me, I just put a wadge of toilet paper in my pants and waited till I got home and spoke to my mum. I don't remember saying anything to my dad or my school friends. Mum was quite matter of fact. She said, "You've reached womanhood."

She used those words?

Yeah, pretty much. She wasn't negative about it, but it was a taboo subject really. She told me, "This is what you need," and she showed me the towels. Tampons definitely were a no, no. It was sanitary towels. And I got on with it. Mum was quite supportive with my pain. When I understood there must be a connection between how I felt the day before and then my bleed, mum was sympathetic with that. Subsequently, every month I would have a terrible time the day before my period came. Quite often I would end up being off school for a day. It was excruciating, really terrible, high temperature, throwing up sometimes, diarrhoea, terrible pain in my back and abdomen. Mum would get me a hot water bottle, and settle me in bed, a hot drink or something. So that was nice. But this continued and I was missing too much school, it was only the first day, but every month it would be the same. It was just so painful, mum got quite concerned. I went to see our GP and was referred to a gynaecologist. They couldn't find anything wrong and put me on the Pill. I was fifteen years old. It was quite a relief really, the pain lessened.

Yes, of course, because you don't have a real period taking the Pill. It's a false period.

Yeah, exactly.

And what you know now, that resting before your bleed and during your bleed can help reduce pain or discomfort. Was that suggested to you?

God no!

Taking you back again to the first time you bled. Do you have any recollection of that moment, did you feel the blood come, or did you go to the loo and you saw the blood? How was the actual moment?

I felt something happening inside and I felt wet in my knickers. I went to the loo to find out was going on and found the blood. There was a warm sensation and then a slight lessening of pain as it started to flow. I don't remember anything other than that.

Can you recall your response to seeing the blood? You knew what it was?

I think it explained why I was feeling so rough. I thought, 'Oh it must be connected to this. There's nothing majorly wrong with me.' So, it was a relief in a way. I was a bit worried. I thought, 'Oh, is this going to be every month (the pain)?'

How much did you know about your menstrual cycle?

We had sex education at school. We were told roughly what to expect, so it wasn't a shock to me. I started quite late. There must have been some discussion with friends at school, I don't really remember. I just took it as a matter of course. I did feel it was a bit late, I was behind everyone. So, in a way I was relieved, it's a bit late but here's this transition everyone else seems to be experiencing around me.

Was it a conversation you had with your friends? Did you talk with each other about your cycle?

I don't remember it. We probably did.

Do you recall any bitchiness about it?

No, not at all.

What about things like PE?

I often used to think up until I started my period, that other girls' boobs were growing, they were developing quicker than me. It's all a bit vague apart from that.

Relating it back to when you started going out with boys, having your menstrual cycle, not feeling ready for some of the sexual advances that were being made toward you. If you had your period, would you still go out with a boy, would you say to him 'I don't want to do this because I have my period?'

That depended on if I had been going out with someone for a while. I certainly wouldn't say anything to someone I just met. If there was any opportunity to be alone, I might say something if I knew him well enough or I was put in that situation. If I had my period, I would definitely say.

Did you feel comfortable about those conversations with a boy?

With my first true love, he didn't make any sexual advance on me. I think that was due to the fact that his father worked with my dad, so he was probably instructed 'Don't you dare do anything!' I was totally head over heels in love with him. He was the most amazing kisser that I've ever experienced – three quarters of an hour for one kiss – head over heels in love. It never actually came up in conversation with him. Then after that, I was yes, more verbal.

How did you manage your menstruating years and how has that impacted on you in relation to The Menopause?

Well, I guess because I had so much pain, I was looking at being menopausal as a future relief from that pain.

When did you start thinking that?

Goodness knows. I wasn't looking forward to it as such, but I knew eventually it would stop the pain.

Did you know that as a teenager?

I don't know. I knew it wouldn't be forever. It must have been part of the sex education that we had at school. The number of years you might be fertile and bleeding. It wasn't something that I feared.

When you started taking the Pill, did the pain then stop?

It greatly diminished. It really managed it. But then I started getting other symptoms. Excessive bloating, I put on weight, getting Candida, I didn't know these symptoms were connected to taking the Pill. Really putting on weight, which I didn't like. I just didn't connect it with that and having the relief of not having that excruciating pain.

As you moved through your teenage years into your twenties and thirties, becoming a woman in the world, independent of mother, father, family; did you then have a relationship with your cycle? Did you chart it, were you aware of the cycle?

I did, pretty much.

Did you do that in a way that was just factual, because with the Pill it's always regular. Or were you charting your cycle in a deeper way. Were you connecting to how you felt in the different phases of your cycle?

Yes, I was actually. I knew that the week before my period I was definitely over emotional. That made me more aware of when I was due. I could link the emotional feelings to my period coming. I was easier on myself, trying not to get too stressed, to avoid doing too much at that time.

So, there was a level of consciousness to your cycle?

Yes, there was.

Did you stay on the Pill over those years and beyond?

Yes, I did.

Was there a time when you thought, I want to come off the Pill because of the side effects?

I didn't connect those symptoms to the Pill. The medical profession doesn't recognise Candida.

Your GP didn't give you any information about the symptoms?

No, goodness no, not my GP. But I'd made some discoveries of my own. I realised I wasn't good with wheat, but that was much later when I already had Fibromyalgia, aged 29. I'd become highly sensitive to all sorts of things. When I got Fibromyalgia, I took myself off the Pill. I started looking into the side effects of the Pill – the medical profession doesn't recognise Candida (as a side effect) – so how would I connect the two? I changed my diet – I realised I needed to eat more protein. I was craving sugar with the lead up to my period. I learnt that what my body actually needed was protein. I learnt a lot in the first few years of getting Fibromyalgia. How to manage my period, and the time leading up to it. I was staggered to find out that the painkiller I'd been prescribed all those years for my period pain, actually had caffeine in it, which makes pain worse! What?! That really shocked me.

So, you were being prescribed the Pill to alleviate the pain, and on top of that you were given a painkiller?

Yes, that's what was recommended.

But it actually exacerbated the pain?

Well, yeah. When I found out caffeine does the opposite to what I was led to believe, I thought, 'Why would they do that?'

How does that make you feel? I can see your anger still in that. So, can you say a little bit about that? Or a lot, whatever needs to be said!

I don't know how to voice it really. Why would they make a pill that would actually make the symptoms of pain worse? Caffeine actually causes contractions and makes them worse. I thought, 'Is this coming from a male's perspective?' It rattled me.

I think this is such an important aspect to be voiced.

Yes, particularly with my own experiences of having caffeine, I learnt to avoid tea and coffee in the days running up to my period.

And then you were unknowingly taking the prescribed medicine that made things worse for you?

Yeah. The Pill and the painkillers combined were bizarre.

I took myself off the Pill in the first few years of having Fibromyalgia. During that time I was quite ill, but also learning so much about my inner world, myself. It was a journey of discovery, not just from a period perspective, but from all aspects.

I'm really interested in this part of your story, discovering you had Fibromyalgia, you made the choice to come off the Pill and you entered that journey of looking inward in terms of what your body needed. Can you say a bit more about that? Was it a purely physical aspect of your health you were looking at or did the spiritual practices come in at that point too?

At that point I had just started to learn about meditation. I was tuning into myself and what my needs were and what wasn't serving me. Self-discovery really, definitely a spiritual aspect. Because there was very little support, I had to have tests done and it actually wasn't for seven years until I was diagnosed with Fibromyalgia. I was just dismissed as having some sort of chronic fatigue syndrome. Because all the tests kept coming back negative, I was just left to get on with it.

This was mainstream medicine?

Yes, mainstream medicine. Although I had great support from a Naturopath Radionics dowser.

How did you discover that?

I can't remember now. No idea, I think it was when I started to search. The good thing in a way, was that the doctors *couldn't* help me, so I took it into my *own* hands and did a lot of research. That was way before you could look things up on Google, on the Internet. It was the library and reading books and actively looking for alternative therapists. I went to see a nutritionist and she recommended the Naturopath and getting snippets and clues from them helped, making sense of things from my perspective. In a way that was positive, I'd taken responsibility for my own health rather than leaving it to the doctors to tell me what to do or what not to do. The first few years of being ill was a real journey of self-discovery.

What age were you through that?

I got ill at 29. For the first four years I was learning to pace myself, learning about the condition and how to manage it. The fourth to the seventh year I was just surviving, treading water and not getting any better. It was in the seventh year I started to make progress. Before that I was stuck, I felt stuck. I really felt this inner calling, an almost primal need to get to the bottom of it, to find out the root cause of the illness, why was I not getting any better? Real soul-searching. And then I found an amazing healer in America and

I had a clearing experience with him.

Was that energy healing?

Yes, energy healing. It was like a regression therapy. That really opened me spiritually and I was able after so many years, to see the light at the end of the tunnel. I realised, 'It's okay, I'm going to get better.' At that point I was actually diagnosed with Fibromyalgia. For me it was just a label. It doesn't really make any difference to me, this word. Because of the soul-searching, I then found my spiritual practice, then got into Reiki and ended up training in Reiki.

The spiritual practice was Heartfulness?

Yes.

When you came off the Pill and you started to menstruate naturally again, how was it at that point?

It was still pretty painful. But I was not having caffeine anymore, which helped, and increasing my protein really helped. I wasn't getting the bloating and the water retention I got when I was on the Pill. So that all helped. I didn't have a great deal of energy, but knowing when to rest and when to exercise in relation to my cycle really helped. I noticed that if I did exercise leading up to my bleed it helped. My circulation flowed better.

What sort of exercise did you do?

Swimming, I loved swimming. It really helped. I also practiced yoga. What also seemed to help with period pain (not during my period but as regular maintenance) was having saunas and the water massage of a jacuzzi, which I did once a week for quite a while.

And on the days you bled, were you in a position where you could rest? Did you allow yourself to take some time out and be still?

It was going to bed earlier. Having longer sleeps helped me. Trying not to arrange too much during those days of starting my period. It wasn't as dramatic as those early days of menstruating, my teenage years. It was less dramatic. I was irritable pre-menstrual but not as it had been, not such a big contrast.

And did you have a heavy flow?

No, never did, it was quite short, four or five days.

And were you aware at that point that during your bleeding days you may have vivid dreams?

Yes, definitely, I did have vivid dreams leading up to bleeding. After the first day, I felt relief, I felt more normal, mentally and emotionally.

And do you feel you had a conscious relationship with your womb?

No, not at all. I think because there was so much else going on, being out of balance, it was just trying to survive for those first seven years. I was trying to balance my whole system. When I was thinking about this aspect, I thought maybe that fighting for survival is a very masculine energy. Maybe that's why I was less conscious of my feminine energy.

What were your expectations of being a menopausal woman?

Well, having seen what my mum went through, it gave me some idea. She was very, very irritable and flew off the handle. When she was going through The Menopause, she was completely neurotic, it was so heightened. It was a more mental, emotional reaction from her that I noticed. Through my therapist training, I studied The Menopause a little bit. I had some ideas and clues about possible symptoms. So, when I did start to get symptoms, I tied it in to being menopausal.

So, how it was for your mother, how you witnessed what that was for her, you used the word 'neurotic' as your observation of her behaviour and what you learnt through your therapy training was about symptoms? So, those experiences are all quite medical model, typical messages and information that we've always been given. The belief that a woman is becoming 'neurotic' because she is expressing the intensity of her experience. Was there anything along the way that said to you, that actually The Menopause is an alchemical transition? That you are going through an initiation of transformation, was there anything that gave you that message?

Partially, there was a sense of a celebration of a transition, a celebration of not having a period anymore. A freedom from it. It was a long time ago, I stopped bleeding in 2005/6. I was 45 when I became perimenopausal.

Was your mum that age too when she became perimenopausal?

She was two or three years later than that. But I have read those women who don't have children, which I don't, often have menopause sooner. Initially, I wondered if it was stress related because I was very busy with work.

It was also the time I emigrated to Turkey, so there was a lot of work to be done, lots of decision making and my periods began to drop off. I thought I was perimenopausal, and I was. When we moved over to Turkey, my periods came back for about nine months before they tailed off over six months and then they stopped. My first hot flush completely took me by surprise. I was in India, in my ashram in deep meditation and all of a sudden, this huge heat came over me. What did I think?

It was an acceptance of it at that point, but I didn't actually know what it was, because it was the first one. It completely consumed me, even though I was in a very deep spiritual space it was quite difficult to just stay put with it and not pull off all my clothes. I just sat with it and experienced it. I can't honestly remember any other details.

I know you chose to take HRT because the hot flushes were really challenging to you. How long did you have them before you started taking HRT?

Quite a long time. It wasn't until 2010, so about four or five years. I tried alternative things. The worst symptom for me was not being able to sleep. I knew I wasn't stressed at the time but because of the underlying problem of Fibromyalgia, I tried Black Cohosh and other herbal remedies.

Not sleeping, hot flushes, off the scale irritability – it was just awful. Looking back, it was like I was acting like a 'mad woman.' I would flip at the slightest little thing; I remember I dropped a bottle of wine coming back from the supermarket and it was like the end of the world. I completely overreacted, it made me realise just what a heightened irritable state that I got into and I had to do something about it. It was horrible living with myself let alone anyone else having to live with me.

Some therapist friends had suggested Black Cohosh. It did help but wasn't the full answer. It made the symptoms bearable by about forty percent, so I continued with that for a while.

Were there any other women around you who were experiencing their changes, that you could talk with, share practices and support each other?

No, I was in Turkey at that time. I would come back to the UK every few months and do treatment swaps with my therapist friends. But no. I was very much on my own with it. I did have one English friend, whose mother was ninety, and my friend told me her mother was still getting hot flushes in her nineties. Apart from that, I don't remember many discussions about The Menopause. Most of my friends were younger and weren't at that stage in their lives. I think I was a slightly lower than average age to be perimenopausal, so not a lot of emotional support.

How about your relationship with your partner? Was it something you talked about with him? Did he understand what was going on for you?

God yeah, especially when I was getting ratty. What really changed our relationship was unfortunately, I couldn't bear to be touched because I was just so hot. We were living in a hot climate. We were used to cuddling in bed in the UK and when we were sitting down relaxing, but I couldn't tolerate it. I think he found that quite difficult. He certainly knew I was going through it because I was just, 'Leave me alone, I'm too hot!' It was a difficult transition for both if us in that respect.

That leads nicely into the next question about how you felt at that time and how you feel in relation to your sexuality and sex as a post-menopausal woman. How do you feel about those issues at this stage in your life?

Not good. Because I would get too hot really quickly and I was irritable, so my body was on alert I suppose. And also, I had a dry vagina, sex was very uncomfortable, that very soon became an issue for me. I didn't lose my libido dramatically at that time, but it was uncomfortable so the frequency was less. It was a negative transition in that respect, thank goodness my partner showed a lot of patience. As time went on, it actually got worse because as my energy levels dropped my libido dropped. For all of those reasons I ended up deciding to go on HRT. For all of those reasons, it wasn't fair on my partner either.

I'm wondering then, when you went on HRT therapy, how much of an improvement was there in relation to the hot flushes and your libido and your relationship?

Pretty big. Definitely the hot flushes reduced dramatically and I was sleeping like a baby. It was such a relief, it really was. So, I was more refreshed, less irritable, it was like I got my life back. Sex was easier and more enjoyable. It had quite a dramatic effect. But, after about 18 months I started to get pain in my liver and I had to take myself off it because I felt so rough. Eventually I managed to get an appointment for an ultrasound. But by then, whatever the drugs were doing, the side effects were too much for me to handle, for my liver to handle. I had to come off HRT and was off it for about two or three years. In the mean time I tried different things like progesterone cream. That didn't work. I tried Sage – that made the hot flushes worse. Then I went onto Agnus Castus (a herbal supplement), which had a soothing effect but no way near the effectiveness of HRT. But it did calm the hot flushes down.

What was your day-to-day life like at that time? I'm wondering were you able to respond to your body's needs in terms of saying e.g. 'I'm going to go and rest now. I'm going to stop being busy. I'm going to stop doing and I'm going to rest'? What was your situation in relation to being able to do those things or not?

It was very difficult at that point. When I was in Turkey, I wasn't working most of the time, so I could rest. But when we came back to the UK, in 2010, my dad died literally just a few weeks before we came back. We moved in with my mum because she had Alzheimer's.

So, I had mum with me, I was looking after her. I couldn't take my eyes off her for more than ten minutes at a time. She was pretty full of energy. From eight in the morning until bedtime, about eight o'clock, it was pretty full on. When she wasn't there, she went to an art class a couple of times a week for a few hours, I started seeing clients. Life was very, very stressful for all of us. Life was unpredictable for all of us. It was very difficult to take time off and rest.

It's interesting isn't it, that at the age we become menopausal our parents can become more dependent upon us? That they become less able to care for themselves and we are called to care for them. Whether it's actually in person, or emotionally via the telephone. Suddenly we're required to be in the role of carers to our parents at the very time when what we really need is space and rest.

So, you've described what has been challenging or difficult during your changes, have there been any aspects of The Menopause that you've felt, 'Yeah, this feels good'? As a woman who has walked towards being post-menopausal, being Crone which you are now, were there any moments when you felt, 'This is actually something else, this feels good'?

That's a hard question to answer because the Fibromyalgia symptoms have just got worse and worse. I would say the only positive benefits as in physical, is not having PMT and period pains, which were always terrible. Yes, I felt more balanced throughout the month, so long as I took herbal supplements, so it was nice to enjoy that freedom from my cycle. But actually, as The Menopause went on, my health has deteriorated, so I can't say I'm celebrating it. I've come to realise that because my adrenals were so shot, and with looking after my mum which was extremely stressful, I was stressed a lot and my poor adrenals were over working when my ovaries were producing less and less oestrogen. Over time my hormone system has become more and more out of balance, so I can't say anything positive about it.

I wonder then, you are a deeply spiritual woman, you have your Heartfulness meditation which you've been doing for over 20 years. Tell me about that.

Yup, 24 years.

I think acceptance is key. I go through periods of rising above what's going on in my body and not getting frustrated. Just getting on with it is how I've dealt with it. There have been times, especially when I have been deeply spiritually connected, a part of me of course wants to be well and there is a drive in me to get well no matter what, versus accepting it and letting go of attachment to outcome. The determination to get better is strong. It's a play between the two. Seeing my condition, menopausal symptoms and the Fibromyalgia, it can be a spiritual insight. If we have perfect health, no money worries, we won't grow. I fully understand and appreciate that to have a health problem helps me to spiritually grow. It helps me to accept what is going on. Without pain we just kind of carry on contented and we don't really soul-search. I feel very strongly that it helps me to stay connected. I'm on the path, I'm accepting the pain because it will help me to grow spiritually.

Second interview one year later

When you look in the mirror now, what do you see?

I see a much softer woman than I was. More connected to myself and to earth, especially now I am living in this beautiful place (West Wales). I see an older woman, but I also see my passion for life inside, that love for life, a real sense of peace and love. I'm happy to be in my body, feeling that peace. When I look back at where I was, how I felt as a youngster, up and down all the time, I'm much more content, more in harmony, more comfortable in my skin. At one with myself, I would say.

I did want to ask you, in relation to the beauty of the place you live in and no longer having your cycle (for a long time) do you feel more attuned to nature's cycles and the phases of the moon? Do you feel differently during the changing seasons and moon phases?

I have to say, with the moon I don't make a conscious note, but I often don't sleep when there's a full moon. So I'll experience something and then I take note of the moon phase. With regard to seasons, I am more in tune, especially now, being a gardener.

I'm a sun lover. I need a lot of light, but I do enjoy the winter because it's a time of rest. In the middle of summer when it gets light early, dark late, sometimes I think 'Oh, if only I could have a few nights of winter time.' I tend to sleep more heavily in winter because there's more time to rest. I love the summer but there is something to be said about conserving energy and rest in the winter.

Leading up to springtime is a time of preparation and thought and planning. I really feel that sense of a promise of new life in spring. I feel a strong urge to be outside in the summer, I look for things to do. Even if I'm exhausted, I want to be outside.

Autumn, I enjoy more now than I used to. I had bad memories from September time, so it was always something that I thought, 'Oh dear, here it comes.' I love the colours of autumn. Every season I enjoy really. When we lived in Turkey, I missed the changes of the seasons, they don't happen over there as it does here.

But winter is hard to manage here because of the cold. It's the first time in years this year (2020 during Covid lockdown) that I haven't been away to get some heat during our winter months.

So, is there anything more that needs to be said about being a Crone?

I feel more settled in myself. That's it. More settled.

Thank you so much Jenny. It has been an honour to hear your story, I know what you have shared will resonate for so many other women.

Reflective Questions

What resonated with you from Jenny's story?

What insights have you gleaned?

What is your biggest takeaway?

LOUISA

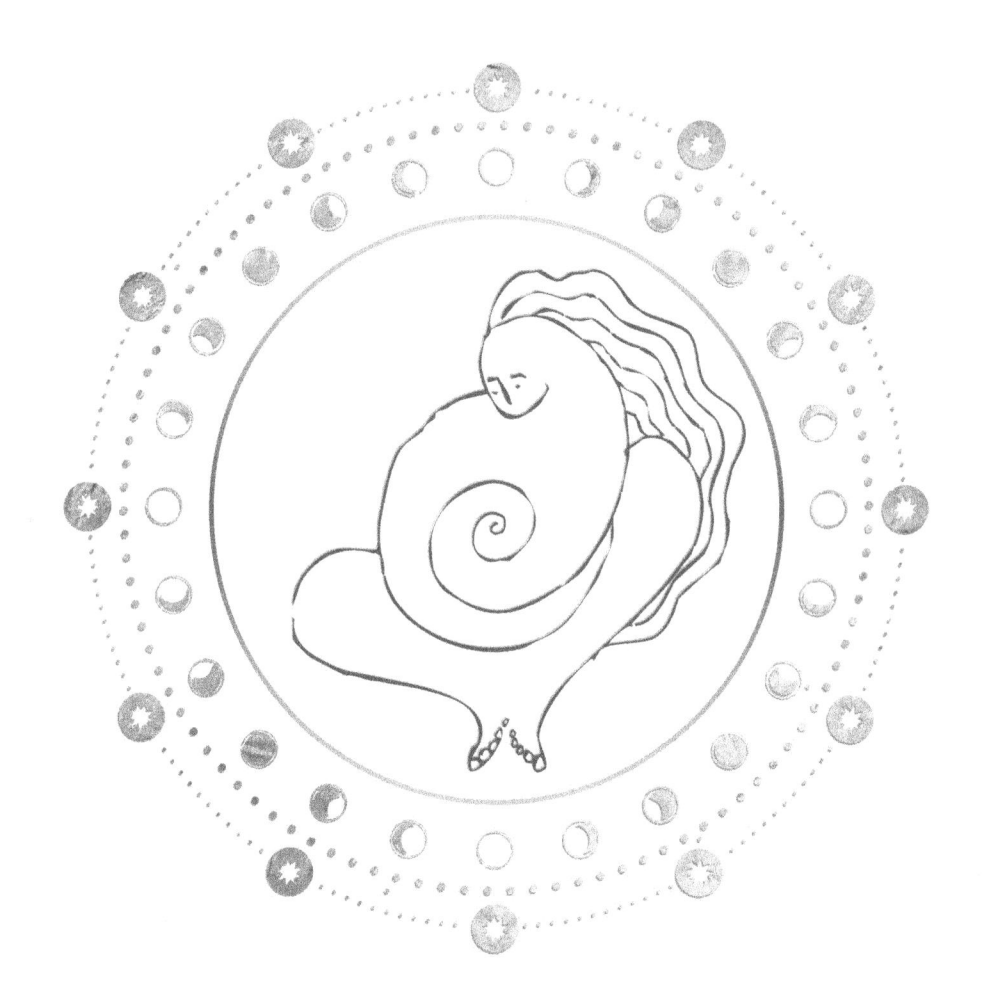

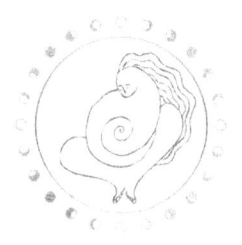

What have you been told or taught about what it is to be a woman? – Thinking back to the first messages you were given from your mother, father, friends and media.

I don't remember particularly being surrounded by strong women. My grandmother was quite a character. She was quite dominating. She had a strong energy, but it was controlling, I guess. My mother's energy I experienced as quite submissive, weak was the word that came to mind really. My mother was diagnosed, well showed symptoms of MS (multiple sclerosis) in her pregnancy with my brother. So, from an early age I experienced her energy as weak, weak in her body because of her MS symptoms. I always experienced my mum as needing to be cared for. That was my experience of my mother, what was reflected back. She was the woman closest to me. I didn't have a sister, I had a brother, and then interestingly, through my dad's reflection, it was something similar. I noticed when my daughter was born and he first saw her, it was a very different reaction to when I had my son. It was like, the feminine is weak, it needs caring for, it needs rescuing. So that was the main theme.

And also, from the male point of view, through my dad, there was very much a thing about the way a woman was supposed to look. I don't remember a lot of praise growing up as a child. For my dad it was what you look like, the dress. There was always a bit of a battle. My mum, she was pretty easy going about what we wore, she was quite laid back. But he liked to see me in a dress – that 'innocent feminine' he liked.

He really struggled when I became a teenager. I felt almost a disgust from him. That was the feeling. I was no longer his pretty little girl. He really struggled with me becoming a woman. That's what I felt from my father.

And my mum was non-descript. She was unsure about her femininity. That was the reflection I got from her. So, that was immediate family. My grandmother passed when I was about twelve.

And then of course you've got friends, peer groups and media, and it was very much a concentration I remember in teenage years, of what you looked like, because that seed had been planted in childhood, 'looking nice for daddy', or rebelling against it. Teenage years for me as a female, was felt through the eyes of that male gaze of patriarchy. Of your body having to look a particular way, doing the face and make-up. That influenced me a lot through my teenage years.

So, being a woman was what you looked like. And there was something there about caring, caring for others. I always felt that responsibility towards my mum, to care for her and my dad in a way. Being a woman was being a carer and the way you looked. They were the main themes when I felt into that question.

And it was sad really. I was almost looking for another mother, as if I didn't have one. I think I was always looking and searching for other qualities of being mothered, or a role model, but they weren't there. I don't think I ever found that strong energy I was looking for in other women.

What was your perception of yourself as a child and teenager?

Not great! When I think of being a child, because I'm a girl and a sensitive child, I didn't feel strong in myself. But particularly I think, the teenage years are always quite revealing. I guess what showed itself in my teenage years was how I felt about myself as a woman, which was not great. Not that I'd rather be a man, but feeling it's pretty shit being a woman. It was hard work. It was as if I always had to try to get approval through the way I looked and that went through into adulthood. So, there was this thing of what other people think and how other people view me. The feeling is, 'Shit, yeah, that was hard work.'

I just wanted to be myself and that for me is happening now!

Where do you feel you are in relation to your initiation?

Physically, the symptoms have been around for years, but mild symptoms. And my cycle is really regular. I would say psychologically and spiritually, I'm definitely perimenopausal. For some reason I put fifty on it, but not like I'll be out the other side of it. But that for me feels like a real transition point. Maybe I've just made that up, but that feels like a huge point.

I don't know whether I've made it a big thing because of other transitions in my life. Whether it's been into menarche or into motherhood, those transitions weren't well supported. There was no consciousness of what was going on. The Menopause is huge for me. This is like, 'Yeah, I can be conscious of this transition.' And there are women around me, like yourself, people that are going through it, that are role models. So, it's really exciting. It feels like I'm definitely in the lead up to something. I feel strong.

Do you feel that's shifting your perception of self? Is it impacting on how you show up in the world?

Yeah, definitely. I don't want to hear what other people think. I'm looking at my body, and it's changed a lot. I can't control that, which is great. I know some women do, but to me that's alien now. Why would I try and cover up the grey? I might choose to dye my hair as part of my expression – I'm not saying no to that – but for the first time in my life I'm not too worried about the look.

That witness that looks and criticises in a way that society says 'I should look,' that's fading. And for me that's a relief and definitely changes how I feel. I feel more positive about myself, my true nature. It's as if my skin is getting thinner, I feel more porous and I can shine through more. And I trust that and listen to that. I've never felt that in my life. In some ways you could say that's sad, getting to being nearly fifty. If I live to a hundred that's another fifty years of feeling good and being actually able to share my gifts!

There is a huge self-doubt. It's as if I wear a little cloud of self-doubt. Not just who am I, but what am I here to share? A saboteur comes out, but I can feel that fading, dissolving more, there's a strength, there's a foundation.

My whole energy structure feels more stable. Some people are just born with that, and just have that naturally, but I don't feel that I had that. Maybe it is through my own mothering that I can build on that. That feels empowering. I know now that I can hold that. And although I've understood that, before now, I just couldn't, I didn't feel strong enough. But there's a strength now beginning to grow in this period of my life and it's lovely, to feel that I can hold myself and hold those vulnerable bits of myself. And there is less wanting to try and hold other people's vulnerable bits. Because that's what I've done to feel safe. I held my mum's vulnerable bits, my dad's vulnerable bits and everybody else's. And meanwhile bits of me were just starving and dying in corners. Now, I'm not feeling so drawn to holding other people's vulnerable bits. Now, I know I need to hold space for myself, not in a selfish way but I know it feels necessary. If I don't do this for me now, where am I going to be in a few years? Does that make sense?

Yes, it absolutely does, it makes total sense. It resonates with me very deeply. I love that you're talking about strengthening your foundations and being inward and that it's not a selfish act, it's a wise act. The Menopause is our time to heal our wounds and to be able to step out the other side in our authority and to hold others in a very different way. I learnt that the holding I did for others and not for myself caused depletion and depression. I wasn't giving to myself at all. I've realised that a thread through this book is the act of nurturing and nourishing one's self, how vital that is for us all and particularly during this initiation.

So, let's go to your first bleed and what your memories of that are. And how that experience is impacting on your approach to being menopausal.

Yeah, that's fascinating, to echo that back, that fascinates me at the moment, that the link is huge. I've got a daughter who's just had her first blood, this year, so, she's on her own journey obviously, but that's reflected back even more, of how connected those two things are. It blows my mind, that connection. For me, there's something about our birth as well. There's definitely some pattern. I've felt it through my daughter, her birth, how I experienced her birth, her first period, how that linked. I'm still absorbing all that. I love these things, how we heal through these transitions, nothing's ever lost, that's what I feel like. I feel as if there's an opportunity now with being menopausal.

My first blood was, on the surface, quite non-eventful. I was looking forward to it, I was excited. I wasn't an early starter. There were other girls around me, I had a friend who was older, she'd been bleeding for a couple of years. My mum was quite open. Her Tampax would be in the bathroom. We didn't talk about it in an emotional way. There was a bit of embarrassment talking about periods, but it wasn't a shock, like some women don't know it's going to happen. I'd had a book in primary school talking about the details. A few of my friends started, so I was quite excited.

Interestingly enough though, on the weekend I actually started, my parents were away, so my mum wasn't actually present. I was staying with my godfather and his wife at the time, and she was a bit witchy, a quirky character and the house had a reputation of being haunted. So, I'm in this haunted house, with this witchy step mum type woman, and I was thirteen. So, it's got that air of being supernatural.

When I started there wasn't lots of blood. I was quite disappointed really, it was like brown kind of blood. I thought, 'Oh, well, I've started,' and I got some cramps. I didn't tell her it was my first period. What came in for me at that age, which is what I've got to address now, is feeling 'the victim.'

I played on, 'Oh my tummy's hurting,' and she responded with the motherly care I was looking for at the time. I don't remember feeling at the time, 'Oh, god, my mum's missed it.' I didn't feel that. I thought, 'Oh I've got a bad tummy,'

And she said, 'Are you alright?'

She gave me a Paracetamol and I thought, 'Oh this is alright, I'm getting a bit of attention now.' That's probably a pattern that's played out, a victim pattern, the mothering I was obviously lacking in and needed.

My first bleed lasted for a couple of days and by the time mum got back on the Sunday night, it had stopped. I remember my mum was in the bath, I went in and I told her. She said, 'Ohhh, my baby's not a baby anymore. You've got your period. Oh, I missed it,' and 'You know where the pads are.' And that was it.

It's so amazing talking about this now, that's how my birth was. I talked to mum about it. On the surface it was, 'Oh it was great. We went into hospital, you were out in a couple of hours.' And it was all great on one level and I got my period and it was fine. But wow, when I've gone into my birth, there was loads more going on. As I'm talking to you now, it's amazing. I'm feeling a similar thing of, 'That's my life, really.' On the surface it's, 'Everything is fine. It's all good; Your birth was good,' and 'Oh my first period was all good,' but to me, I feel it in my heart, I feel sad.

Can you say something about what that sadness is?

Sad that there wasn't a depth of something else, of nurturing and care that I needed. Whether that was at my birth, or my first period, I needed more than what was expressed. I needed. That's what's come in as I'm talking. I can feel the emotions, that's only now as I'm talking to you, I can feel the connection of it all sounded fine, it was all described as being fine, there was nothing bad, no trauma, and my mind says, 'Well that's all fine.' But it was what was missing. And that's just as valuable. Wow, that's really interesting! And that's coming in now because I'm strong enough, I can hold all those bits.

How do you feel that is filtering in?

Since my daughter turned twelve, I have felt my Maiden-self closer and I can hold her with strength, instead of the victim part holding her. Like with my baby-self saying, 'Please, help me, somebody help me,' and wanting someone outside to do it, which never happened. I'm grateful for that now, because I have to show up. I've got to be gentle on myself. It's only now that I'm ready to do that. I can feel my Maiden-self close enough now, and I can give her what she needs. I'm lucky that my children are old enough that they need me in a different way, so I can throw myself into that more. I can reserve enough energy to hold that, and my baby-self, my new born self.

Growing up with my family, there was this whole surface thing going on, but the undercurrent was totally different. There was a split. I feel now in our family, it's okay, especially when the mother is the centre of it all. I'm able to say, 'You haven't done anything wrong, but at the moment I'm just a bit touchy.' I allow myself to be like that. For my family to witness it and feel it. It gives them permission as well and the reflection off everybody at the moment is beautiful to see, everyone is healing. I've been more allowing of that. There was a protective layer I think, because it brings up the emotions that are uncomfortable to feel. I'm sure it's a part of The Menopause, this transition. There's an opportunity to take that layer off and feel it and see all the gifts. Not just for myself, but for the family. That excites me, and I feel it. It is challenging, it is uncomfortable, but what I'm seeing in all the family is a gift. I sometimes see my mum and dad and think, 'Wow, have they changed, have I changed?' There's something that's shifted.

I'm becoming more comfortable to be myself, and they're more allowing of that. Or maybe they always were, and I was keeping myself a prisoner, I don't know. But all the reflections are, 'It's okay to be Louisa,' to be myself, feeling that acceptance part of me closer.

I've been journeying with the poem The Journey by Mary Oliver. I've played around with that poem for years, but it's only now that I get it – about 'saving the only life that you can save.' But for me and everyone around me, it's not just, 'I'm okay now.' It's my interpretation of gathering all the parts of myself that have been lost, so that I can model that to others, so that is good for others. All these other bits of people, I can say, "Well, actually, that's yours. And whether you're strong enough or not to hold it now, it's not mine to hold."

Not crossing a boundary. And it all goes on in the unseen, but also seeing it physically in family members is healing, it's amazing.

What did your mother and other women around you model to you in relation to The Menopause?

My mum went through it when I was becoming a mum for the first time. So, I was going through a huge transition, and she was going through Menopause, so that's interesting. Again, with my mum, it was on the surface, really like non-eventful. So, I remember it was a bit disturbing, witnessing her as a younger woman. It was as if she and other women lost the plot a bit. Mentally, they seemed a bit unstable and changeable, and that disturbed me a bit – I didn't like that. Previously experiencing my mum as consistent, there must have been a wobble. I noticed that in other women too.

Over the last few years, since I've been journeying with my menstrual cycle consciously, I've been looking forward to The Menopause as an opportunity, knowing it in my bones that it's an opportunity for healing and a conscious transition. Sitting in Circle, being around older women, and seeing the messiness of it, and the gifts, it didn't scare me. That's more recent.

There was a yoga teacher I used to go to. I was in class and then suddenly there was a mental, emotional thing, which bothered me. I didn't feel safe around it. It wasn't huge or traumatic. It was these women around me went a bit weird! Things that *I* do now, like calling people different names, I laugh at it now. But thinking about the question, the part of Menopause which scares me, it's that 'losing my mind.' Losing control over my mental ability, not being able to multi-task. As a younger woman, seeing other women going through their Menopause – who had been capable of doing more than a few things – then witnessing them talking in a way that all of sudden seemed a bit confused. It made me think of deterioration. But it was just temporary, just a blip, and that did happen with my mum.

I don't think she took HRT. But again, my mum doesn't complain. She didn't seem to have a heavy bleed. Neither of us as teenagers had acne or spots or anything, but she got them during her Menopause. And she couldn't go in the sun – her cheeks were quite hot and red, and she was embarrassed about it. It went on for a few years, I remember that. But mood-wise, I don't know what was going on underneath the surface. Outwardly, it didn't scare me watching her go through it. By the time she was fifty, her periods stopped. It was at a point when I had already moved out. Things in her life were settled. So, she modelled, 'Yeah, it's okay.' But it wasn't like an event. She didn't see it in a spiritual way at all.

Is it something you feel drawn to talk about with her now? With your foundations feeling more solid, do you feel able to talk to her about how you are experiencing your changes? How you want to go inward, how you are showing up in the world differently, how you care for others and yourself, setting your boundaries? Are those things you would like to explore with your mother?

No! No, not really, I ask her questions, like what age she was and stuff like that.

I used to ask questions about my birth, once I got on that journey and did some rebirth work, but she was always defensive about that; as if I was going to point the finger and say you did something wrong. With The Menopause, she gets defensive too, as if I'm trying to blame her. So, the desire is not really there to have that conversation. On the surface, she seemed to get through it quite smoothly. But her personality is, 'you don't complain or talk about feelings.'

She's not really in touch with her body, actually. I realised this as I've been really wanting to massage my legs. I'm making oils myself – that's my medicine to rub into my legs.

She's told me she can't sleep at night because she's got restless legs syndrome. I said she could use some of my oil, but she wouldn't do that herself, she'd look for my dad to do it and he probably wouldn't. So, she's more likely to go to the doctors and get some medication. It could be linked to her MS, I don't know.

I see her get confused when I say things like, 'Not being embodied,' or 'Being fully in your body.' She looks at me a bit confused. I think that's her defence. She doesn't feel a lot of her symptoms of MS, because she's not fully in her body. So, what I'm trying to say is, the conversation for me wouldn't be enough, because I don't feel her experience as fully embodied. So, we just have snippets of conversation. But as I do the work, it's all connected with my mum, my daughter. I trust that part of her knows and we communicate on that level and I can feel her looking at me with something that has shifted between us without having the conversation.

Do you feel a connection with your lineage? Or is there a gap, is there a loss?

Both if that's possible. I never thought I'd want to research my family tree, but the more I've concentrated on this work, there was at times a pretty intense, obsessional desire to know more about my grandmothers' maternal line. And that brought up a lot of sadness because I was finding out things my mum didn't know about. When I'm telling her now, she's like, 'Well, they're dead, what's the point?'

The point for me is, I got to fill in the gaps. I found out where the family came from, where they lived. There were some photographs. I felt a leaning into the lineage and what it was about. And it did feel there were definitely patterns. The caring thing was definitely there. My grandmother was a stronger woman, a matriarch. She was a carer, a middle child, she cared for her brother and her parents. Her older sister got to do what she wanted to do. There was a break, I still haven't quite healed that. Something happened, like my mum was the missing link, something like that. I can't quite put my finger on it with those connections as I work back.

It might be a life long journey for me, working back. I feel now the strength of my maternal line. There's a lot of woundedness, and I haven't quite connected yet to what I would call the ancient mothers, and partly that feels something to do with my mother. But there's enough, a foundation, to be able to be connected to the lineage. There's a lot of wounding but there's a lot of gifts, a lot of strength, and I feel that more than ever in my life, like there are cheerleaders saying, 'You're doing it for all of us'. And especially for me, for my daughter. There was one point when she came into my bedroom and said to me, "I know the name of my daughter." And she told me what the name of her daughter would be, and I felt my granddaughter.

Goodness, that's so beautiful.

I do have doubts when I see what's going on, on the planet. And when I talk to Sisters who have a view that extinction is closer than we think, I feel the presence of my unborn granddaughter and I know, whatever reason there is for it coming, that it's worth it.

I know some people are choosing to clear their lineage and end it, and that's fine; for my maternal lineage, I feel that we chose to keep on coming and that gives me strength. Learning about the women who came before me, the babies they lost, the lives that were lost, there's a strength there. It's coming through the lineage, not so much from me reaching out, but that they can touch me – and that feels part of the menopausal journey, that opportunity to do that. And it's not that it's easier, but I can't not go there! It's definitely part of this journey and that connection to our planet, and of course the connection to our bodies, and also the acceptance of 'who knows?' That's another big theme that's come up for me that I've found difficult, *the unknown*. When I let that go. When I just let that go, I think 'okay, the next generation may not be coming,' and I let that go.

I still have hope.

Or do I fall into despair?

It was the plants then that spoke to me. The plants said, "We still need this planet. And we can regenerate it. Even if humans have to go. We need your support now, to do as much as you can. Clean it up. Clean it up. Clean it up. So, we can restore, so that at a future date it's available."

That is so moving. I feel that too, Louisa.

That was the message. And that made me feel more connected to plants, to the planet, and my body. That regeneration, that transformation and the magic of that. And that's hope!

If humans have to take a break from this planet, that's not the end of the world. I mean it's not nice, the process we'll have to go through. That *connection is still there*. I didn't want to disassociate and distract myself from everything that's happened. I still want to stay present with what's happening. Whether we keep on going and there's another generation.

For me in my lineage then, knowing that there's that strength, gives me hope. And gratefulness to my ancestors who came before, when things were difficult. They gave me life, they kept going, they had that survival instinct. And now it feels like they're saying, "Yes, survive and thrive and enjoy it!"

It's a beautiful planet we're on, we're privileged to be here, let's enjoy it, even with the mix of things and the messiness of it all. Just enjoy it. And for me, I feel it's that letting go now, *allowing* myself to have pleasure.

What came up for me as you were talking, was a remembering of something I experienced a lot of in the disintegration phase of my Menopause where I would feel utter despair and complete joy the very same moment! It is the most extraordinary feeling. But I think what I learnt from that is, of course we feel that despair because what is going on in the world is messy and terrible and has devastating consequences. But at the same time, there is such utter, beauty and kindness and exquisiteness in the world; and they are walking along side by side. So, of course we're going to feel them both. And I think that helps us to connect to our ancestors and to Mother Earth in the way you have described.

It's that life line I always look outside myself for, and then I became disappointed because I couldn't grasp anything. For me it felt like, for a lot of my life, like I had an umbilical cord, like a lasso! And I was looking, for something, to attach to. Obviously, there's attachment issues there, going back to my mum, I realise that. But I still had this strong desire for someone to come and rescue me, save me, something to connect to. It was only when I brought that in and felt the lineage, that I began to feel stronger, but it was hard to turn that around.

With being menopausal and whatever changes were going on, that door opened and made that more available.

Second interview one year later

Welcome back Louisa, it's so lovely to see you again. Let's pick up on what you were saying about feeling stronger and doors opening.

I realise talking to you, all those invitations, opportunities of whatever's going on as a menopausal woman are a gift. Before Menopause I would always see black and white, a split of: there's either this or that. And I love now that I can feel and see the beauty and at the same time be almost on my knees in despair. I can feel grief and joy, and I can go, 'Wow!' They're both going on in my brain and my body. That's *new* for me, maybe over the last year or so. I love that, to feel both. It feels like magic to me.

Maybe I have always been able to do that, but for me, even with my menstrual cycle, it was like, 'Oh, yeah, I feel great building up to ovulation.' It was like black and white, then it hit a certain point and 'boof,' it was really tricky then, that change of mood. I don't feel that so much now. It's all in the mix. And I can *hold* that. Maybe that's what it is, I can *hold* that. There's a bigger container. I have strength, I can hold *all* of it. And I feel that getting stronger.

And these are bizarre times (2020 Covid lockdown). I feel I want to be close to people, physically in contact and be held and we're being nudged because we're being told not to. But that's that whole theme, isn't it? The separateness and the togetherness, that polarity is so out there right now.

Yeah. And for me, that's why my shamanic practices are so healing, because the core belief is that we are inseparable. We are all one. We are all Divine. We are never separate from the Divine, from each other, from nature. Mother Earth, nature, has been so nurturing for me throughout these months of lockdown. My heart really reaches out to those who don't have access to nature.

The video you did down by your stream was so beautiful. It warmed my heart, it really touched me in that moment. And I guess that is something we can do for each other, to share something from our life that touches somebody in that way and it can be online. It doesn't always have to be in person.

It was a pleasure to do and to share. It was interesting to me because I had been laying low, dealing with health issues, but as I began to emerge from that and reach out to people again, I felt a connection that was, unsurprisingly, really healing and supportive. There is a danger for us all, that in an enforced isolation we forget to reach out and to say, "I am feeling really low at the moment and I just need other people to know and hold me in their thoughts."

Yeah, exactly.

I think this is really fascinating also in terms of these interviews that I am doing with all of you wonderful women, because of course, when we did the first interviews it was before March. It was before it all kicked off (Covid). None of this was on the radar, we were all just going about my business.

And before I arranged all of the second interviews, I was thinking, 'Goodness me, how must it be feeling for you as a woman going through The Menopause, through your initiation, while also going through this global initiation, the whole world disintegrating as we know it. And we don't yet know, I don't even know if we'll know in our lifetime, how it's going to re-member and reform and reshape.

So, I am really interested to know how it's impacting on you as a menopausal woman?

Yeah. It is funny. I was talking to a friend, we're in a similar kind of place with The Menopause. We check in with each other every now and again. We've been asking "What? How did this happen?" How did we end up, going through this *now*?

Like you said, it's an intense time, being in the menopausal pot and the bigger global pot which also feels menopausal. It's like an end of a cycle initiation; but there is a *gift*. So, part of me, like today, when I am feeling open and optimistic, and awakened, I have a feeling of looking through that lens. It's like, wow, what a *gift* that is, all that reflection is aiding my process. It's supporting my process, intensifying my process, whereas, before I could hide from things I am feeling; I can't hide from anything now, which for me is what this menopausal initiation is. It's in your face, something not resolved is in your face. It's just *there*.

And in these current times, I think everyone is experiencing that. Well, the opportunity is there to look I guess, and see it. Whether we choose to look is another thing, but I *am* choosing to look most of the time. So, in that way, it is the gift. But on more fragile days, I feel, 'What? Did I really choose this? What is this all about?'

At the moment for me, it's a gift and I've cleared the decks. I wasn't committed to any work. I'd recently taken my daughter out of school. I'd not planned anything, I haven't booked anything. Last year was really weird for me, coming up to this year, thinking I've got nothing planned, no work, kid's not in school. But in a way that all meant there was no hassle. I mean, of course finances are a worry, but I gave myself space to experience what's going on. You asked some questions about what is good about Menopause and what is bad? And I was feeling into that, pondering on that for a while, feeling where I am in my menopause journey.

I'm feeling *more*.

I realise that everything is more than just black and white, this or that. Whether it's viewing stuff that is going on in social media and what side people are on or polarities or what's going on within myself.

What I found when I considered what were not so good things about Menopause, of course, there were good things too. It was both. When I looked, I found a balance, I love that.

That is the biggest gift of this whole process, being able to see and feel that it's both, the polarities. It's, win-win in a way, even when it's uncomfortable. What I feel when I say that is the alchemical pot or that sacred container that is Menopause, that is the womb. I haven't experienced that before, although physically my cycle is changing and I am experiencing that differently. My whole body feels like a cauldron of transformation which can hold *more*, it's stronger.

And I guess my boundaries are better. There is a big thing about boundaries and territory. I am finding the moment reflected outside and within myself, which is a positive (as in, to hold myself), but can be the walls of separation as well, between people or between parts of myself. So, I am aware of my blind spots. I'm willing to look at myself and face things. But I'm aware that there are parts I don't look at. A gift for me is interacting with other women; being shown and being willing to look at what's being shown within me.

I'm being gentle with that and not forcing it, because sometimes it is tricky.

Using dreams is really useful at the moment, which helps. This is the time of year when I like to slow down and with two weeks of lockdown, I don't have to worry about Halloween costumes or going out trick or treating. Normally I go on a deep retreat at this time, but there's none of that. It's just like, a clean slate. So, I can just be for a couple of weeks.

That is amazing, Louisa. I have been tingling listening to your words, such clear and powerful insight into the process.

I'd like to pick up on what you said about your working with your dreams. I'd love to hear a bit more about how you are doing that – what you receive through your dreams, how you are using those insights?

I had one last night. It's perfect timing, amazing really, because my dreams are quite mundane usually and last night, I had one that wasn't mundane at all. And I've been sitting with it this morning and I know by just sharing the essence of it now will help me to get more later. So, I really appreciate you witnessing what I am going to say, because I don't really understand it yet.

Sometimes I go to sleep with an intention of dreaming to help something or just to recall. And I didn't last night. My night was quite restless, but I went into a nice sleep this morning. My 'good' dreamtime is if I am up early. Sometimes I go back into a semi-conscious state, which I did this morning.

The dream's theme was that I was on a land that felt like it is where I lived, and I was native to that land. And as far as I could tell, it was *now* but it felt old as well. And there was a feeling that people were coming to invade the land. I think I was with Andy, my husband, and our son and I think the dog was there. It was my current family.

The fear of invasion was there but everyone else was carrying on as normal. And then I felt shock that the invaders were coming quicker than I thought. We had retreated enough that I could look down and I saw people coming in from the sea with guns, coming into the land.

The feeling was that we had enough time to retreat up the hill to get away from them. But it was still a shock.

Down on the land, the dog was still alive and somebody else in the family.

I felt fearful because we couldn't wait for them, we needed to retreat. I hoped they would know where to go. And then there was grappling, you know, that feeling sometimes in the dream where you want to run, but you can't run. I was in grass and I couldn't go quickly enough.

Then we were in our village. The village was like my house, or my parents' house, like modern day times. I felt relief we were there, but knew the invaders were behind.

So, we had to hide, it was a bit like Lord of the Rings. I remember at one point, Andy was there (this makes me quite emotional), Andy covered me to protect me. He had a magic word that made us invisible to the intruders. But the intruders felt familiar at this point. It didn't feel like they were the enemy. At some point, they left and they were going back to their land, and we thought it was all over.

So, the dream had a feeling of fear. I feared the invaders because they didn't know us. We didn't know each other, we were different, from different lands. It was like they were coming back to reclaim what was theirs. And we would defend our land, but there was fear that they could hurt us.

Andy protected me and kept on saying, "Say the magic word." We became invisible. It was amazing to feel the darkness and be invisible. I was trying to hide, but there was nowhere to hide and I felt, 'Oh, where am I going to go?' I just lay on the floor and nobody saw me.

The overall energy was very much that the invaders were coming to our land, but the land was familiar to them too as they went to places that we built as if it were theirs. Part of me felt that I understood but it felt bad as well.

So, it felt like a boundary thing. It could be different timelines, but also what it sang to me was *nobody owns the land*. We are *all* immigrants, being moved around, and I think with the lockdown and especially current times, the restrictions of movement, I am discovering that people are territorial about certain areas that I have lived in my whole life.

The dream feels very current.

Boundaries can be healthy too, creating a sacred space. And what I feel more than anything is, we *all* belong to this earth and who knows who moved where and when and what our ancestry is, so the dream feels ancestral as well.

There's always been cycles of humanity where there's been a fall and maybe we didn't make it as a species. Perhaps we had to leave the planet and leave her fallow to regenerate before we came again. The memories feel as if they still lay within the land. For me, staying connected to the land and the earth and staying embodied is difficult, sometimes I'd rather float away into the stars.

We don't know what lies ahead, it's unknown isn't it? The feeling of the unknown was in the dream as well. It was a good dream, I'll carry on working with it. I'll write in my journal, name it and write a few details down and then leave it – not try and pick at it too much, because then some of the magic goes. But just write a few words down and trust it's informing me in some way in my day-to-day life.

And I know just by being witnessed, it will unfold. The timing is perfect. And I think that's important for me because I felt some depth of magic and a mixing of timelines in my dream last night. That is rare for me. I don't normally get ones like that. So, thank you for asking about dreaming.

Do you remember what the magic word was?

No, it was a totally different type of word. It makes me feel really emotional recalling that part of the dream. It was a totally different tongue. It was a magical word that maybe I am not meant to remember, but also it linked me and my husband in a way that I have not felt before, that he would be willing to risk his life for me.

I think, with our relationship at the moment, sometimes I put myself in the stronger position of protecting *him* like I would a child. Maybe it's a safety thing as a woman, to put myself as the mother. And he allows that a little bit as well. But in the dream, he was the strong one. He was the protector.

It's so interesting actually, as I am saying that, I listened to an interview recently with Alexandra Pope interviewing a couple going through Menopause. And they were talking about how sometimes she took the role as the strong woman but through Menopause, she felt she needed to rest and allow her husband to hold the space and that was in her ancestral line. As far as my maternal line was concerned, I see quite passive women, but for her, it was like a long line of strong women that did not allow men to be equal. She said it felt quite threatening to be vulnerable during Menopause and allow the man to hold space.

That reminded me of the time of my son's birth. It's a time when we are so vulnerable as women. I felt, 'I can do it, I'm strong, I can do it on my own. I can hold my own,' and we don't allow the man to hold space. So, a little part of us has to realise, 'Oh, I need you.' And I think it's because there are certain points in our life cycle as a woman, maybe when we're having a baby and maybe it wasn't planned, in *those* times we may think, 'Oh my God, he could leave us.' And ancestrally, those would have been the times that we really needed the man physically to protect us from predators or invaders. I know with some animals, the female will protect and care for their young, but you know ideally, we need tribe or a partner there.

So maybe the dream has brought all that up! Knowing in the dream that he, Andy, is there and he *is* strong enough to protect me and he has *magical powers*; he has his own intuition. Sometimes he says things and I kind of brush them off, but actually the masculine intuition is amazing and he has his own magical powers – as does my son. And I don't always see that or recognise that or want to see it because there is something a bit scary about allowing that, maybe because I am usually the healer, the counsellor, the one that holds space.

That resonates deeply with me, Louisa. Letting go of being the strong one, the healer, the counsellor, the holding it all together, it's difficult to surrender.

But for me, the moment that I started to do that, I heard the magic of the male perspective, the male intuition as you have described it. Thank you so much for sharing that.

Okay, so what you have just shared about your relationship, flows very beautifully into the next question.

What are your feelings about your sexuality and sex as you journey through Menopause?

That is such an interesting one because I would say definitely for the last couple of years physically, we haven't been particularly sexual.

In the past, guaranteed around ovulation, or sometimes bleeding time or just before, I felt very sexual. It's interesting now, I have been feeling into it, because I get the hormonal thing that happens at ovulation, but it's different.

So, in the past, if we have not been sexual for a while, chances are my hormones would take over at ovulation and that would be the window when we get that connection and it's all good. But that's been changing recently. The desire isn't just a given.

We've both had to get used to that, which was difficult, I think, for Andy initially. But then we fall into periods where he is not interested and I'm not bothered. And we are like, 'Oh shit, we're going to have to put some work into this.'

What happened before sometimes, is we would connect by talking and making time and space for connection, then naturally we would want to connect, not all the time and not always with sex. It's making space or having a time for that.

He's out working all day and sometimes it's so easy to do our separate things. It's important to make space for that time of connection, feeling intimate and then naturally wanting to be physical with each other. That *has* changed for me.

I mean, my body has changed, so when we have been making love, I've had to stop him a few times. We just have to get used to this as well.

Before Menopause, it would just be full on, the body just takes over and it's just hot. That's not there anymore.

It's so subtle what's going on and it feels different to me. It's obviously still there for him. I can feel it in his body. I want to explore it, you know, like slow it down and notice how it feels different.

How I feel about my body and my sexuality has definitely changed and I'm getting used to that. It's quite nice, after being a woman that was very critical of her body. I quite like that my boobs are saggy and I don't have to wear a bra and my skin is like softer, I feel more through my skin.

So, there's that transition of the hormones changing – I'm not getting that high sex drive anymore. I am talking with Andy about him coming into my space, letting him know my boundaries are important. Before Menopause, I think he could come into my space and it would not bother me, so he could touch me on my breasts or whatever. Now though, I'm kind of more, 'Oh God, that was too quick, you can't just come into my space and put your hand there.' And then he feels rejected and he pulls back, and then we have times when he feels scared to touch.

We've had times when he is waiting for *me* to initiate it, and then *I* think, 'Does *he* still find *me* sexually attractive?' I know he always has, that is one thing about me and Andy, is that he finds me physically attractive, whether I believe it or not is another thing.

So, we've had that whole dance going on. But that feels as if it's getting easier. It's taken a couple of years but there is an understanding now.

I think his body is different too. There was a *neediness* before, like in bed in the morning, that's not my time really to feel like connecting in that way, and I would feel a neediness of him needing something from me. That used to feel a bit icky – that's how the energy felt to me. And we had to go through conversations about what that was about, which was difficult for me to express and difficult for him too. He felt rejected and hurt. He thought I was saying I don't want him physically, but it wasn't that. It could have been old stuff or some kind of shadow masculine energy that I felt wanted something from me, but it just felt icky.

So, we've had those kinds of conversations and I'm feeling quite comfortable in my own skin. I'm really grateful that he's given me space, not put pressure on me for sex or for our sex life to be back the way it was. And although it has been uncomfortable, I'm quite excited that, as long as we put in the work or the time to be intimate, we can carry on. It's just going to be different.

It's just how we relate sexually; it's just going to be really different. But it feels as if it could be deeper and more sensual, a whole-body experience rather than just our genitals taking over and being hot and going for it. And that kind of peak experience, it feels like it can just be a slow burner, to be mindful of it. I can see how it could be quite easy just to shut all that off and just not even go there. When the desire is not there at all and you think God – it's been months now!

We had a joke the other night, 'Should we just check that everything is working?' And I thought, 'Well, it might not work and that's another thing I can feel uncomfortable about. Can we actually start the process?' I think, 'What if I can't do it anymore?'

It's okay though. You know, we can both stop if one of us is not feeling it, whereas in our younger days, oh my God, that would have been really frustrating and would have caused issues between us. So, actually, as I express this to you, it's quite beautiful what we experience now as a couple and how I feel about my body sexually. It still feels sensual.

I have started making and using body oil. I make an oil and then massage my body; I've been doing breast massage recently. Sometimes it can be more yoni massage, or even anal massage, which can be really, really grounding, especially in these times, for the root chakra. I did tear there during my son's birth, so there's maybe some scar tissue. I remember massaging, leading up to the birth, the perineum, using oil. And then it was not something I've done for a long while. It really brings me back into my body, not like a sexual feeling, it's more sensual. I go really deep into the breast and find bits, not lumps, I'm not scared of that, finding something.

I guess it's a good practice if you did have something, you would know if something has changed. But it's amazing. God, and my mouth, it just amazed me the bits that I can get into and my cheek around my jaw where I must hold a lot of tension. The oils and massage are a soothing practice that I would not be without through this particular transition.

These are such gems, Louisa. It's so interesting to hear the different practices you are each developing and creating for your wellbeing.

Massage and oils are definitely my favourite.

So, you've started to talk about how you feel your connection to your womb and yoni is for you now, through your wonderful practice of massage; connecting to your feelings around your sexuality and your relationship with your husband at the moment. Is there anything that you want to add about how you feel connected or not to your womb and yoni?

It is, for me, and always has been, a work in process. I think that's why I'm always drawn to this kind of work. I listen to other people talk and it's like, 'Wow, they really know their cycle.' I've been following my cycle and interested in this work for quite a few years now. I still have moments where

I don't feel connected. The tracking I do, I feel embodied and grounded, and to me, that is womb in a way.

How do you feel when you look in the mirror now and how do you feel about being a woman as you walk ever closer to becoming Crone?

When I look in the mirror now, I feel I can give myself permission to just be me. Especially when I reflect, like the last couple days, looking at photographs of me in my younger days.

In those days, I felt an outside pressure, that I put on myself. It took a lot of energy. Not that I was into the latest fashion or whatever, but I believed you *have* to wear a bra, you *have* to put your face on to go to work and look a particular way. And I didn't realise I was caught up in that until I reflected back and look at photographs and go, 'God'! It just took up energy that I haven't got now. I would rather put that energy into this process.

Of course, there are days when I look at my skin, for example. It's always been quite thin and now it's even thinner and it's more of a concern. If I see little red spots, I think, 'Is that fragile? Is it *too* fragile?'

What I'm trying to say is, it's not so much a concern about what I *look* like to the outside world. It's more like, 'Oh, is that normal? Is that okay?' I'm not quite fifty and I wonder if I'm going to be around 'till I'm eighty. Will my skin get so fragile that I'll bruise really easy? So, when I look, I may notice things that are to do with getting older and think more about my health than what I look like to the outside world. I am more comfortable in my own skin, which is good.

It's funny, it's like the word 'Crone,' that still feels like a long way off for me. The Crone energy is around me but I feel like I'm between worlds, in that transition. I'm still bleeding, but I don't feel menstruation like I did. That is a big one for me. I don't feel fertile. I think that's what I'm trying to say, I'm still bleeding and my cycle is quite regular. I could go on bleeding for years, but it's not the same. It's different. I can't even imagine what it must be like to *not* be bleeding. I'm getting used to being in that in-between world. I can't even give it a name. I'm not Mother, I'm not Crone.

I'm feeling my Maiden more. Maybe that's to do with having a thirteen-year-old daughter. But you know, the veil is thin now, remembering what it was like to be pre-puberty and not bleeding. And that excites me, remembering. I could feel the emotion rising when I talk about her (the Maiden me). I'd forgotten her. I lost her for a while. I'm allowing myself to reach out to her more and in my dreams.

Being around my daughter I notice that transition for *her*, when the hormones change, women become more equipped for motherhood. And again, depending on your ancestral lineage or other things, sometimes that can take over. Motherhood really grounded me. Now, I feel as if I am transitioning to an age where maybe I can tap into more of my Maiden self. So that is quite exciting. I never really got the full cycle thing before, but I'm kind of getting it now. It's being in the unknown. All of it is in the mix. If I could see through the unknown darkness, there is a bright Maiden there, who is even whispering to me now, of hope. And you know, what those years of wisdom bring feels lovely, because it's got the whole life experience. The Maiden with all her life experience. She is in the distance just there. She is like a bright little light.

I feel the Maiden, the Child, is such an important piece right now, because I think all of us have forgotten so much of what that was. We had innocence and we were connected to our intuition and our insight and we knew how to play spontaneously. We conversed with the fairies and the trees and we felt it all with such ease as children, that springtime. I think reconnecting to that is a big piece for us all because it's that lens of joy and wildness, isn't it? Seeing the beauty without the stuff that starts to come in for us as women when we start to bleed. If we are not held or nurtured and nourished to stay connected to our Maiden self, to know that is always a part of us, we slowly, over time, lose sight of her. But as you say, one of the gifts of The Menopause is that we remember to invite her back in.

Yeah. To be free and to be wild again, It's something about that wildness. I can feel how it's coming through for me. I've always loved animals; I can feel that coming in stronger. And that is from my Maiden, my younger self. She loved animals. There are two sides to that. There's a shadow side that sometimes I would rather be with the animals than people. So, there's a heightened feeling that I would love to run away into the woods with a load of animals or become one of those women that have got a cat sanctuary. There is a temptation from the shadow side of escaping with the animals. They are my friends, because I trust them but I don't trust people.

There's also a connection that I see them as family.

Our family cat recently had an accident and he had his leg removed. It was very shamanic. There was talk about dismemberment coming up even before that happened. He showed our family something and there was some gift in that and he is fine. Some days I do want to just stick the leg back on. It brings up something about my childhood of wanting everything to be perfect. There is something in me that doesn't like illness or death or disability. It scared me, his accident.

And it brings back again, my childhood experiences, that when things around me were different I felt uncomfortable. My daughter is really different. She seems to be okay and more comfortable with difference. But for me as a child, I don't know why it was a threat. So, anything different triggers me. A child having a temper tantrum would scare me or somebody who was different, not as a prejudice, it just scared me. Sometimes we are just scared because it is different.

So having a young cat lose his leg was scary. He's still beautiful, not perfect. Beautiful. But that perfection thing and holding on to that, Menopause is definitely gathering my fragments. I'm getting out the nitty gritty parts of myself that feel repulsive and ugly. Now, I'm being encouraged by reflection of people outside and things that happen inside myself to realise, actually, that is part of me.

There is also a fierce part of me, a part that might hurt people. It's not part of a good, nice girl. And those parts need me more than ever now. I'm looking at how I can build a bridge or work with those parts?

A whole new conversation about astrology has come back into my life, in a new way by working with the myths and the archetypes, a more feminine way of looking at astrology. I have dabbled a bit with astrology for years and all of a sudden, it's coming back this year in a totally different way, a more ancient astrology.

A part of me knows that working with the ancient feminine archetypes is helping me access parts of myself I have not allowed before, like the savage woman in me, the one who is willing to kill. And that brings up the death mother and the shadow mother and all those parts, the shadow bits, that we would rather not look at. So that feels like a big part of Menopause for me. I don't want to miss that opportunity. Because otherwise it's just going to bite me. I know it's uncomfortable, because I feel a bit of shame. It's like an outside voice of being shamed. And it might be from other lifetimes, the witch or the intuition that came through and being told, 'That's rubbish.' When I am aware of internally shaming myself, I have a word with that part of myself, I tell her, 'You cannot do that anymore.' It's quite messy, but at least it's moving, connected and embodied. Perfect. Yeah.

Thank you so much, Louisa, it has been an absolute honour to hear your wisdom and your insights, your dreams and visioning. Thank you.

Well, thank you for listening. I think it was perfect timing today, I am really grateful. I have realised that there isn't a map for The Menopause, nobody prepares you for this journey. And even when you do the work, nobody's got a map! You create your own. I realised that just little things that people say, just a little guiding light supports you on your way.

Reflective Questions

What resonated with you from Louisa's story?

What insights have you gleaned?

What is your biggest takeaway?

MAGGIE

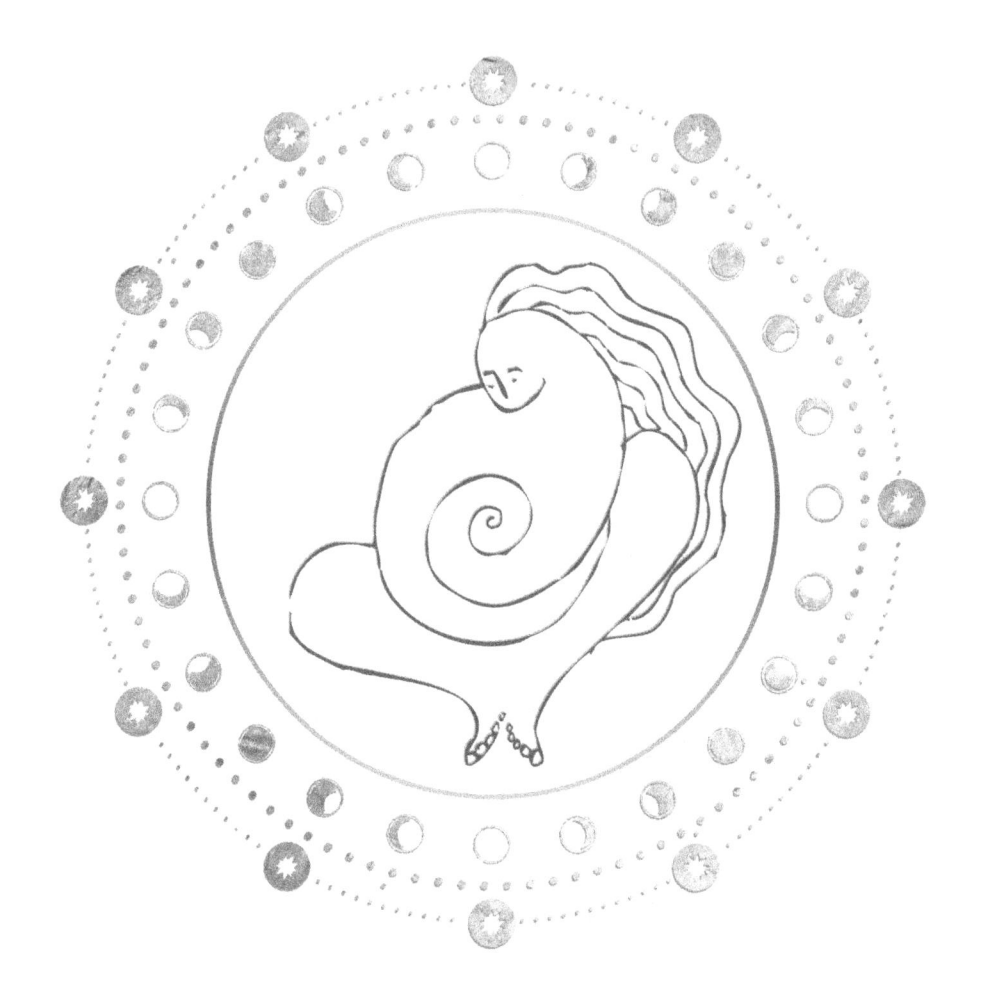

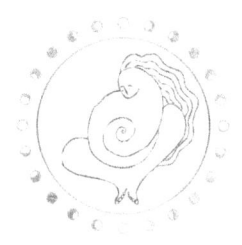

What have you been told or taught about what it is to be a woman?

I wanted to be a boy. I loved being mistaken for a boy in Scotland when they called me 'sonny.' I had very short hair. I played with the boys a lot, so I probably had messages, but I don't remember overt messages as a child.

My mum left several times, so there was a sense of loneliness and isolation. At one point we lived with my father's uncle and aunt. The uncle was abusive, so that was more of the message I suppose – that being a girl is dangerous. Being a boy had more autonomy, more agency.

I was quite a wild girl/boy as a child. Then we moved to London, my mum and me. Dad joined us later. I think puberty was a shock, and it wasn't long after that the pressure started, especially for my generation, to lose my virginity. I lost my virginity to, seriously, an 'Irish Ponce.' He had all these women out on the game. I refused to go on the game, so I suppose I held out there. So, I had mixed messages.

My mum adored me and my dad. They loved me, my parents, but they were going through a difficult time. There was a lot of deceit because they were trying to protect me but I knew something wasn't right.

I think I had this thing that a lot of my generation had, which was, you are either a good girl or a whore. If you lost your virginity before marriage, you were a whore. I lost my virginity at fifteen. It was a very alienating experience. It was the first and probably the only time I've been honest. When it was over, I went, "Was that it?!" Because I'd read all these girl magazines about fireworks, crashing waves, that sort of thing. I was waiting for some sort of transcendental experience.

I was fifteen when I started working at the Windmill (a club in London's Soho district). We had to wear all this make-up. I had Boot's theatrical removing cream – I remember Mambo Jo (the man I lost my virginity to) putting cream all over my body. I lied about being a virgin to my flatmates because the other girls weren't, nobody else was a virgin! Our generation was so different to now, or maybe it isn't. The circles I move in now are very different to the one's I grew up in.

I remember I put a note on the door in the flat I shared with these other women, 'Do not disturb, I'm having trade tonight,' and of course Mambo Jo didn't believe that I was a virgin. I was terrified, all this cream was going on, and it just happened and it was really a let-down.

And then later on, one of my flatmates was obsessed with jazz. I hated jazz, but because I loved her, I pretended to like jazz and I got a crush on a jazz musician and then fell in love with jazz. And then I began to realise just how low status it was to be a woman. I mean I did already, but this was more reinforcement. I didn't see a single woman playing an instrument. I thought women were biologically unsuited to play an instrument. Some women sang, which is why I became a singer. I suppose I used my voice like an instrument. That was my way to try and capture some of the music that inspired me.

So, all the messages I got, all the books, everything, was by men. You assumed doctors were men, scientists were men, painters were men – that was the message pre feminism. I forget sometimes just how bleak it was. It didn't mean there weren't strong women around, there were. So there were some role models and that was mainly in the arts.

I started going to 'Ronnie Scott's' club when I was nineteen, Ronnie's club. The *music* saved me. I was treated like shit – there were predators and they really preyed on me. I was very naïve. I wanted to talk about the music and they thought, 'Oh, I'm in there.' I was romantically carried away by the music and thought, 'Oh, I have to talk to that beautiful musician,' and they took it as getting sexual favours, so I was an unpaid prostitute.

It was at Ronnie Scott's that I met Denis, who mentored me and wanted nothing in exchange. I started finding some self-respect; he really mentored my singing. There were some strong women there too in theatre. My boyfriend, who became my husband, used to tell me that feminists hated God, and I was into God, so I was terrified of feminists! I was in the canteen of the Oval House and there was this book by Germaine Greer, 'The Female Eunuch,' and I remember thinking it was a 'dirty' book. I borrowed it. I don't remember much about it, but there was a chapter that stood out for me. I think it was called 'Fear and Loathing,' it was all about girls and women and sexual exploitation – and it was like, 'Whoa! I'm not a stupid scrubber!' The personal *is* political. And that was an incredible revelation, so I'm very grateful to that book. And then I came across socialist politics, and at first, they were a bit hostile. They said feminism was a diversion from the class struggle. So, I got plunged into socialist politics and didn't come to feminism until 1977 when I got a crush on a lesbian in a play I saw, I was doing workshops at the same venue.

My daughter was born in 1970, so I didn't have the best messages to pass on to her either. And then when I did get involved in the Women's Liberation Movement, then of course everything changed. I was a born-again feminist! My poor daughter wanted to wear dresses and I insisted she wore dungarees.

So, up to Women's Liberation, the messages I got were not good. My mum believed passionately in me. She ran away from home – she was orphaned. She wanted me to be a performer. She always made me feel that I was a genius. My dad was more strict. I've always had that strange cultural mix, of my dad being Scottish and my mum half Berber, half French

How did those polar opposite attitudes from your parents and the messages and experiences you had as a young woman impact on you as you travelled your womanhood?

I was just desperate for men's approval until the Women's Liberation Movement, which was transformative. That's when I started enjoying other women's company and not to talk about boys because that's all I had ever really talked about to be honest. You know – what crushes we had and what heartbreak. So, my transition from girl to woman was pretty consistent with being low status – girls and women being low status. If we were adored by a man or approved of by a man, then all was well. The Women's Liberation came after I had transitioned from girl to woman. So that was when my awakening came and I thought, 'Actually it's great to be a woman!' I'll never forget my first 'women only space.'

They were very mixed scenes where I went. Previously to feminism being in my life, I went down the West End clubs. It was a butch fem' scene, working girls, the thieves, the hustlers, lesbian, gay, straight – everybody mixed in the underground scene. A policeman picked me up once from a club and told my dad, "Your daughter is mixing with the scum of the earth, the dregs of humanity."

But they were like family to me. The musicians were the ones who treated me badly. The villains were quite old fashioned. The Women's Liberation did heal quite a lot of stuff, not everything. The wounds I got have never gone but I've transmuted them creatively and they're part of who I am. And you can't re-write history but what I can do is have a different perspective. I did the things I did so I could get into the club. It was all about the music, I sacrificed parts of myself for the music. When Denis mentored me, I got my self-respect through the music – creativity and being around people who started to accept me as a musician rather than as somebody to be preyed on.

So, I transitioned from being the prey, to one of the 'boys' or a comrade. Once they recognised my ability as a singer, then I went through a period where I wanted to be different from other women. This was before feminism. Female singers were really not welcomed, unless you were Billie Holiday or Ella Fitzgerald, someone really with status.

How old were you at this time?

This was when I was about sixteen or seventeen years old. I started at The Windmill when I was fifteen, as a dancer, and then I sang in a strip club in Manchester when I was sixteen. And then the feminism came in, in my twenties. My daughter was born in 1970, so before I found feminism. It was after her birth I was exposed to feminism. And then I plunged into relationships with women, having huge crushes on women. I don't do things by halves; I've been celibate for the last twenty years!

What are your memories of your first bleed? How old were you?

Just that it was a bit of a shock. But to be fair, I was thirteen, my mother called it 'your little red friends,' which I thought was nice. But because my mum had been going away, I was quite hostile to her. I was angry with her when she went away to see this other man. So, good messages from her about my blood and just generally really. My mum absolutely 'bigged me up,' she always has, my beautiful, beautiful mum. With my peers, it was always the 'Curse'! And I much more listened to them. but it's good that I got that other message from my mum. I mean I remember it now, so it was obviously a positive reference.

That's so lovely. And in terms of your cycle, how did you experience the different phases of your cycle? Was it something that was taught to you, or did you discover it for yourself?

No, it was never explained to me. I think I used to get quite tearful, feeling quite paranoid – that was my PMT. I got cramps sometimes. If mum did talk to me about it, I don't remember. I remember 'little red friends' but I don't remember anyone giving me any information.

Is it something you talked about with your girlfriends at school?

No, I just got on with it.

Do you remember the moment, the day you started to bleed?

It was more, 'Oh, what's that?'

It's strange, I just can't remember. I do know my mum reassured me. I can't fault my mum on that, she was lovely, but I don't remember her talking about pre-menstrual tension or anything like that.

Did you know it was going to happen, that at some point you would start menstruating?

I don't remember! I can't remember, maybe. I probably must have known, because other girls must have had their periods. Maybe I was waiting – thirteen is quite late. Maybe I was thinking, 'Where is it?' I have a vague memory that I was waiting. But the age thirteen, for some reason, I do remember.

And of course it was a difficult time around that age because mum kept leaving dad. She'd leave, come back, leave again. So, I didn't have my mum around. I stayed with my dad. I couldn't talk to my dad about anything, so that probably was quite difficult.

Did you feel you needed to hide your pads and your cycle from your dad?

Yeah, 'tough guy,' yeah.

Do you think your experience of your menstrual cycle impacted on you at all as you became menopausal?

I think luckily, I found the 'Goddess women.' It wasn't something feminism addressed very much until women like Monica Sjöö. To be honest they were seen as the 'lunatic fringe' because all the other feminists were talking about economics and sexuality, sexual politics. And the Goddess was seen as a bit loopy. But luckily before my periods stopped, I was exposed to that and started to embrace loving my blood. And it was like, 'Oh no, I've just started to love my blood, all these possibilities of ritual – oh no, now it's gone'! So, in a strange sort of way, I'm very lucky that I reframed my attitude towards my blood. I'd even had a menstrual sponge for a while, which was great. I did hope no-one would come into the bathroom if I was washing my sponge! I'm glad that I had a little bit of time, loving my blood and calling it my blood, being aware of the sacred nature of it. So I'm very grateful to all the Goddess women.

That's so interesting to hear Maggie. It's exactly what happened for me too. Just when my bleeding became irregular, the Goddess came in, the sacredness, my blood, all of that. I used a sponge too – what a game-changer! How old were you when you stopped bleeding?

Around about fifty-one, fifty-two.

And did you know what to expect as you began your transition into Menopause?

The only thing I knew about was hot flushes. I'd already been exposed to herbalism, stuff like that, so I knew I wasn't going to have HRT. I knew a medical herbalist who said make a pot of sage. Make it hot, let it cool down, and if you get hot flushes in the night, just drink the cooled tea. And it was brilliant!

Oh, I haven't heard of using cold sage tea for hot flushes! That's great to hear.

Yeah, it was brilliant. So, yes, I got hot flushes and they were uncomfortable but I think because I was around women who had a whole different concept of the Menopause to the usual, it made such a difference to my experience.

Were you here in Wales by that point?

Not long after, I came here in 2002, I was fifty in 1998, so just after. I knew about my Saturn return. My first Saturn return was really powerful but I didn't know what it was. There's something about being aware of cycles that really allows you to go through them in a very different way. I remember I was seeing a healer around here; I was going through quite a depression at my second Saturn return, and she said, 'Sometimes depression is a herald of things to come.'

I never forget that.

As you say, that disintegration, it was all around my Menopause, post-menopause time. It was very deep. Again, thanks to women like Monica Sjöö, I learnt to reclaim the dark. I'm in love with the dark, the sacred dark. I get quite protective of it. When I hear it being demonised, I find myself going, 'The dark is sacred. Where would the seeds be if it wasn't for the nurturing sacred dark?' I'm always on the ready to do battle on behalf of the dark.

I get so saddened about how the dark has been demonised. It's all 'love and light.' I have nothing against the light, I love the light, I just want equal status.

I find it fascinating too. Now I'm post-menopausal I've also reclaimed the dark. It's such a beautiful place to be in, the visioning and the dreaming, the stillness and the connection to the earth – which as you say, is where all life comes from.

Mmm, yes, the womb, we come from the dark and we return to the dark.

Exactly, and I think that's one reason why the dark gets demonised, because the womb is the power of women.

Light and dark are neutral, in nature they are dancing partners, they're beautiful. But the way that we project as a society, Buddhism, all the religions – it's all about banishing the dark – 'Don't go to the darkness,' 'Light a flame.' No!

It's so powerful isn't it because people think, 'I've got to be happy, light and bright,' all the time. And of course for women, within our menstrual cycle we're naturally invited to go into the dark. We find an inner fierceness that invites us to cut through the crap – and that powerful insight has also been banished. We've been taught to ignore our cyclical magic, just get on with it, don't talk about our blood or our insights or our potency. Our cyclical nature is powerful!

It is powerful, yes. I think a problem with our society is that there's not enough dark. It's all light, screens, computers, television. We're told we have to produce, be productive. And then we crash into the dark, rather than melt, and be in the dark, be nurtured by the dark. I always feel the dark mother is a beautiful dark being, that has been and still is abused. But she says, 'I'm still here and I love you anyway.'

But of course, if you exclude something enough, people will have a negative attitude towards the excluded. So, then we have the sacrificial dark mother, but we have the vengeful dark mother too, see what happens if you exile me!

Absolutely. I think that is the rage that many of us experience during our menopausal years, we begin to say, 'I'm not going to banish the dark anymore! I'm going to reclaim it all!' We stand in our power and our sovereignty.

It's great. In music, it's so ironic that all of a sudden there were all these people who heard of how I founded, with another woman, The Feminist Improvising Group. And all of a sudden there were all these young women wanting to know the history, and all these academics were coming to me because I'm an elder. It's definitely something about being an elder.

Now, in wider society, older women are very much invisible, but if you are lucky enough to actually have been involved in some sort of field and you survived being in that field, as you get older all of a sudden it's, 'Oh, I've become a legend!' It's bizarre, I'm a legend in the music field! So, in a way, there is something quite lovely about being an elder. My hallmark was that through my improvisation, my whole life would come out. I revealed my vulnerability. That was really frowned upon, it was seen as vulgar. But *now*, it's seen as something really good because I'm *old*! I have a status as an older person in the arts.

And this is what we need.

Yes, it's good for younger women to see that too. I think younger women are so happy to *see* elder women, whatever we're doing. I remember when I thought thirty was old. I was at the Oval House – one of the women in the fringe theatre who was thirty – I remember thinking, 'Oh, it's okay to get to that age!'

We elder women who are now the role models for the younger women, is so different to my experience of being a younger woman when the only role models were women bound up in the patriarchy. The young women who sit in my Circles blow me away. They are so connected to their cycle. They're working with their blood and the dark, doing ritual and have an appetite to talk with us, the elders, and to learn from us what is yet to come in their life cycle. We didn't have that.

What I was told about the Menopause was that it was a horrendous thing. It was going to be unbearable, or if you didn't have HRT, it would be a disaster. I think the nocebo is as powerful as the placebo. If you're told enough about that, I can see why a lot of women would opt for HRT and I know women who say they've been helped by it. I think because I had been exposed to alternative messages about the Menopause, the wisdom and the rebirth, the Crone, my experience was totally different. I remember a friend telling me she'd been to the Glastonbury Goddess Festival, and was introduced to the fourth female archetype – the Queen (or Enchantress), so we have Maiden, Mother, Queen, Crone. That thing of Menopause is a time of power, made a difference to how I experienced the Menopause. I'm absolutely convinced of that.

Yes, me too. That's why I'm excited to be sharing all the stories here to paint a fuller picture of the Menopause. And of course, what we are saying won't resonate for all women, but I know too, there will be women who will have a sharp intake of breath moment and feel a deep sense of relief. I was that woman.

There was feminist literature I had, for which I am so grateful. Before that, it was just an attitude of, 'You're dried up and that's it.' That thing of being dried up and barren, that your only function was to have been reproductive. Once you're no longer reproductive, that's it, that's the end of you.

Do you recall your mother's experience of the menopause?

No, she never shared anything with me. But I do know she suffered a lot of depression. I could have asked her – why did I never ask her? I *could* have asked her. I didn't know anything about my mum's periods or Menopause, it's just not something we ever spoke about. It's weird, I wish I had. I don't know how old she was when she started Menopause. Maybe some of her depressions were when she was menopausal.

Were there any aspects of the Menopause you disliked?

Not really, no. I didn't even mind the hot flushes, I really didn't. I mean sometimes they were a bit 'Whoa!' But it was okay, I knew I could just make a sage tea and that worked a treat. I think I had a good Menopause.

From what you've said it sounds like you enjoyed the transformation and what it was bringing you.

Yes, because I was already deeply into ceremony and ritual, paganism and the goddess and witches. Once I had come across all that, everything changed for me.

Yeah, I get that.

So, when you look in the mirror, if you do, what do you see?

I'm learning to love what I see. I still can feel, 'Oh no look at all that saggy skin.' I do still dye my hair. When I was younger and first went grey, I just let myself turn grey. But I still haven't shaken off those feelings of, 'Oh no!' I hope by the time I'm eighty or ninety I'll be a bit more accepting. Mum dyed her hair until she was probably in her eighties, even nineties. The one thing I got from mum was, she hated the fact that age defined people. Although there was a paranoia in it, there was also a wisdom in it. She hated sayings like, 'Oh at my age.' She would not tolerate that. She was ageless in many ways, an extraordinary woman, everyone adored her.

Earlier you touched on how you feel now about your sexuality and having been celibate for twenty years. How is that for you?

For fifteen years I identified as a lesbian, although I still got the odd crush on men if there were no women around. I was always looking to fall in love, it was a bit of an addiction. I suppose it was a search for redemption because of all the degrading experiences I had. So, I was looking for the one that would heal the wounds.

I was having a stable, wonderful relationship with a woman when I was singing in Berlin. She was a mentor in many ways. She was younger than me, but she was very stable. She'd done martial arts since the age of seven, so, when I had my rages, she wasn't afraid of them! I was frightened of them; other people were frightened of them. But she was strong and for me it meant I could let everything out. She could handle anything. She was *amazing* for me.

I began to realise, because I had crushes on men too, that I was probably bi-sexual and that felt a bit scary. Because patriarchy said, 'All she needed was a good man,' I felt like I was betraying my sisters. I was fighting a whole part of myself. So, after my long-term relationship I had a few shorter ones with men and then I sort of drifted into celibacy. I haven't been with anyone now for probably over twenty years. It feels fine, it actually feels really great. There was a younger man I was attracted to and he to me, but I felt it was just not a good place to go to. I thought, 'Is this going to be nourishing? Is this going to be healthy? Is this going to be a mature relationship that is actually going to be part of growth? Or will there be arguments and difficulties all the time and be exhausting?' And for *all* the passion in the world, I don't want *that*. I'd much rather be on my own.

I enjoy being on my own. That's quite interesting. It doesn't mean I'm not open to something, but no, it's good.

And do you feel connected to your womb energy?

Well, that's a strange sort of mix. I was in therapy for a long time – my womb is my safe space, it's where it can also be quite dead because of the sexual exploitation. It's a double thing. It's my place of power and it's also my place of almost disassociation. And that's strange, because anything I feel, my womb is the one place I never feel any fear. I've had images of blue lagoons, beautiful fertile places. But also, I sometimes feel like it's just not there, so it's very contradictory. I could probably do with reclaiming it in some way.

I've grown to understand and love myself sexually, which has been fantastic, much better than almost anything I've experienced with anybody. I think I still have quite distorted sort of fantasies because of certain things that happened to me. I think what I would really love to do is find a group that explores sexuality in a different way, that is something I am really hungry for, maybe a woman's group, somewhere I can feel safe to really talk freely. I still feel quite vulnerable, quite ashamed, quite ambivalent about my sexuality. I'd like to reclaim the sacred nature of my sexuality. There's been a couple of butch women who, because they didn't experience exploitative situations with men, they had an unselfconscious wholehearted raunchiness. They were able to be raunchy without it being twisted, and I thought 'Wow, that's what I really want.' It was this wholehearted love of sex and sexuality, without it having to be taboo or dirty. I think we've been quite damaged as a culture through patriarchy. On the one hand it's puritanism and the other hand real exploitation, violence.

There's a younger woman I know who wants to take me out shopping to get a vibrator! I'm going, 'Oh no, oh no!' These young women, they're amazing, it's no big deal! They just enjoy sex, and I'm going, 'Oh my god, I can't go shopping for a vibrator, I'm too old'! She's amazing.

There's an amazing young woman I know who is so comfortable with her blood, her sexuality. Talking about what she desires, she writes wonderful posts about the joy of orgasms, whether it's with herself or a partner.

Oh wow, how old is she?

She's twenty-three!

That gives me great hope.

Absolutely, the connection between those young women and we elders is so rich, the weaving and the learning from each other. We can heal our old wounding from hearing, learning from their unboundedness, but a safe unboundedness.

Yes! They're not about to be exploited, they have agency. I do remember even back in my days, there were a couple of women who had agency and they were the ones who were called the slags. We were called slags even if we didn't have agency, but I remember there was such a double standard and women weren't supposed to enjoy sex.

I need to reclaim my sexuality.

Goodness, so we're at the final question.

How do you feel about being a woman now you are Crone?

I love being a woman, I still feel I'm in my Queen energy. I love, well probably mixed feelings, my immediate response, my true deep, heartfelt, womb-related response is YES! The socialised, wounded part is frightened of aging, I really get frightened. There's someone I used to get really hostile to, because I misunderstood her when I first became a feminist, and that's

Louise Hay. I've since learnt a lot more about her and realise what an incredible woman she was – all the work she did with AIDS and self-love. And I love that she started to learn to play the piano aged eighty! She was absolutely, vehemently passionate about women being able to dress how they want at any age.

And mum too was a great role model.

I had a rib injury recently, someone fell on me during a contact improvisation, and it's still quite bruised. If I have anything that's physically debilitating, then sometimes the more pessimistic thoughts kick in and the fear of getting old. You know, as I'm awakening, I don't want to be 'past it'! I love programmes about elders who are still being sexual. I need more exposure to the fact that when you're older you can still have a full, active sexual life, if you want.

Somehow, the sense that you're ugly with age gets to me. I used to tell mum how beautiful she was, and she would say, 'Oh, no, no, no.' There is that thing that if we don't have flawless skin, we're no longer beautiful. Even though, I can look at other women and see their beauty. I can think, 'Oh you're gorgeous,' but when it's me I think, 'Oh, no you're old.'

I absolutely agree. I wonder if it's because we've grown up with ourselves, we've looked in the mirror all our lives – I still expect to see a much younger me when I look in the mirror.

Yes! I feel so young and sometimes depending on the mirror, I'll look and think, 'Oh you look great,' and other times I look and think, 'Oh my god, you really are seventy-one. Jesus you're old!'

I pull my skin back around my eyes and chin and think, 'Oh I look thirty again like that'!

Yes, I do that! I think, 'Oh dear, look it's all sagging!'

I'm so grateful to all the women who have gone before and all the women who have been pioneers and those that have been invisible, all the women who have been magnificent in their own right even if we've never known about them, all the women who have suffered under patriarchy, all the women who refuse to be brow beaten. It's quite extraordinary really.

I was asked to do a reunion of the feminist improvising group, and I said,

"Well, we don't exist anymore. A couple of the women no longer play instruments, the woman who founded it, she died."

We were going to be called The Women's Improvising Group, and the organisers, Music for Socialism, they called us The Feminist Improvising Group. So, I thought we could call ourselves, at last, The Women's Improvising Group. We had five women from Europe and five women from Brazil. Towards the end of the first gig, they all looked to me as the elder. It was an extraordinary experience. I found these tears of joy and remembrance, 'Oh yes, women, singing with other women.'

Playing music with other women saved my life. I'd almost forgotten, I just take it for granted now. I work with loads of women in music. But having ten of us together, I could remember when I was the only woman. Seeing these younger, amazing women is wonderful but we cannot take for granted our liberation. There are still young women and girls self-harming, hating their bodies because of the messages they're given.

So, we must remember, we need each other.

I love that Maggie, remembering we need each other. It has been an honour to hear your richly textured life experiences and how they are leading you to becoming Crone. Thank you Maggie.

Reflective Questions

What resonated with you from Maggie's story?

What insights have you gleaned?

What is your biggest takeaway?

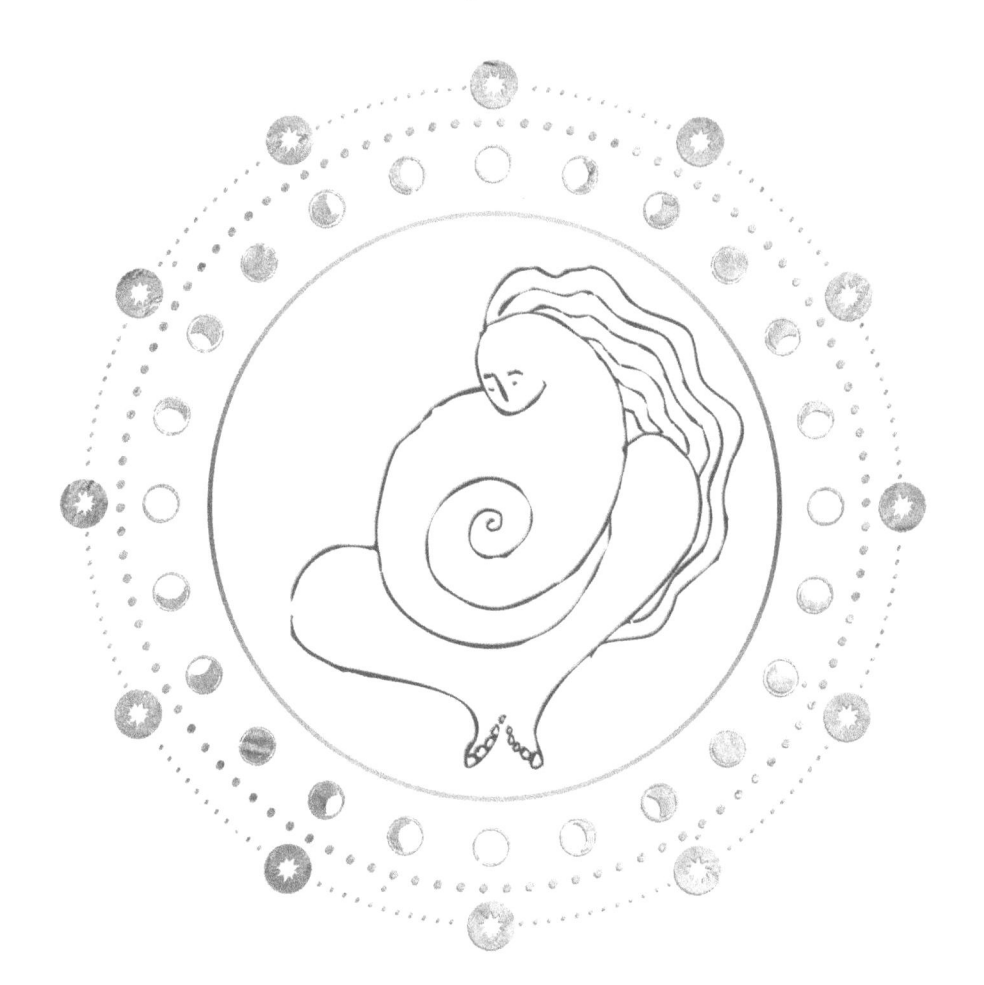

MEG

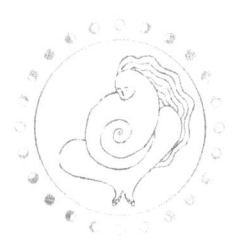

What have you been told or taught about what it is to be a woman? Think back to the first messages you were given from your mother, father, friends and media.

Generally, I feel like, from an early age, I was programmed. The program was to help me to fit into a society and a culture and to give up my own wildness and to deny that and think of it as wrong. The details of that involve all kinds of things, like how to act, how to value things, how to value myself, how to relate to people. I mean it's so complicated.

But, personally for me, my mother had a very bold and confident and empowered personality. But she behaved in a way, in a world, that did not match that all the time, which was confusing. Her role, which she seemed to celebrate and she really, really trained me to also have a similar role, was almost as a servant, to support the breadwinner – husband – it was almost like we were workers in a system, that we were supposed to give up our individuality in a way. And I totally swallowed it, hook, line and sinker. I was such a good girl! I could set a beautiful table, I can cook amazing meals, I know how to clean. I received a lot of praise for these things and I sublimated myself, completely – just like my mother did.

I shouldn't say completely though.

I learned about motherhood from my mother, which is part of what I was being trained to do. A woman is supposed to be a mother, without question, that was almost just automatic. Luckily, my parents also wanted me to become educated, so I did go to college. And yet, everything about the way I was raised, including about how they approached college, was very different to my brothers, which doesn't seem fair. But it is what it is.

The way college was approached was that my brothers had to think about what they were going to study in a different way than I did. Because, I 'would have a husband.' It didn't really matter what I studied. I could just do really what I wanted – which is good – but the reasoning behind that is sort of faulty, because I wouldn't have to be the bread winner, or so they thought. Then there's all kinds of other things like, I didn't have a middle name at birth. My parents didn't give me a middle name, but they did give family middle names to my brothers. This has always felt problematic, since I was a little girl, the reason behind it, which they share and they're very comfortable with it. They're not ashamed of this decision at all. They're proud of it almost. So, their reason was that women take their husband's name and then their maiden name becomes the middle name. And these are the sorts of things – being raised as a woman – I was set up to not be a whole authentic individual, all on my own two feet. I was to exist in relation to other people, always, with a role attached to that as 'supporter.'

The other big part that I learned later was that I was not to act entitled and not to feel entitled and almost that entitlement was something to be ashamed of, like 'don't puff yourself up,' 'don't feel too important.' These kinds of things were synonymous with things like 'misbehaving' or 'being inappropriate.'

Did those messages come from both your mother and your father?

That's a good question. I always think of it coming from my mother. For some reason, she was a much, much stronger influence on me, both because she had that personality – I've even used the metaphor 'bulldozer' to describe her. She was incredibly dominant, domineering in her personality, not in her role! I learned things from my father that my mother could not teach me. He was, is, both of them are still living, he is more of a dreamer.

His centre is emotional. He might not like that he's emotional, I don't know, but I learned about emotional things more from my father. He cries, I don't think I've ever seen my mother cry. And so, in some ways, I think he may have been reluctant about his role in this kind of system. I don't think he enjoyed being the breadwinner, the primary breadwinner, but I don't think he questioned it at all. I don't think for him, there was any question at all that this was his role. His parents were very hard on him and so he didn't think he had any other choice, that's clear. He also had mental health issues – they taught me a lot about how the family system is supposed to operate and it's not necessarily the healthiest model. Which is, we deny our personal individuality, whatever it is we're going through, apart from what it is supposed to be, we push that aside, we don't talk about it. And my mum was very strong, healthy, she would pick up the pieces both at home, and she ended up basically managing part of my father's business as well – she really took care of him. I am not sure she liked that she was doing that.

My father passed on what he knew and how it's supposed to be. I think that they both over the years, influenced me becoming a woman. I think I have baffled them in many ways.

When did you become aware of these different role models of what was being taught to you, the expectations of what a woman should be? Was it as a child or as a young woman?

So, when did I become aware of being trained to be something that didn't come naturally?

Yes.

That's a good question too………. I don't know when I did. I don't think I could even think about it in that way until maybe when I was going into puberty. Because I depended on them so much for my survival, I don't think I would have questioned what I was being taught. Sometimes I'm even reluctant to share some of this, because it feels like this is part of my training as well, that I feel like I was never allowed. Like I had to think of my family of origin as the 'ideal,' like 'this is a happy childhood.' And it was, in many ways. My parents were doing their best and I had a really good childhood. They were a part of the same system I was a part of and they were teaching me how to survive in that system. I didn't know it was a system or that I didn't belong there, until I started to become individuated from my parents.

I do remember looking in the mirror when I was all alone and seeing my reflection and talking to my reflection as if it was holy. I wrote in my journal from about age ten. It felt like a really safe and sacred place for me to be myself. And I would also write letters to God in my journal. And so, I think through that process, I could be real, I could be 'there.' And I think I did start to realise that I couldn't be 'that way' anywhere else and that I had to hide that away as my own private thoughts. But that didn't really come until I was a teenager. And even then, I still celebrated my family 100%, I didn't question any of it really, maybe a little bit more each year, then a little bit more.

Even now, I'm still uncovering layers. I'm learning about how much of this is actually stored in my *body* – what I'm even conscious of. And some of that – I don't know if the timing of coming into perimenopause is a coincidence or not – I think it's probably not a coincidence. So, I'm realising even now, 'Oh my goodness, this makes so much sense why this is happening.'

Another sort of unique part of this journey for me is that I have hip dysplasia, which is a congenital condition. It was something that was developing for me even before I was born, while I was inside my mother's womb and it's been with me my whole life, I get very emotional when I talk about it.

It's helping me learn about this body, the storage of some of these issues in my body, and through my hip and trying to heal my hip and heal this emotion that comes up whenever I talk about my hip. I'm realising it and it's a blessing and it's really amazing to keep uncovering layers.

I love what you are saying here Meg, I was smiling when you were posing that question to yourself, 'Is this a coincidence or is this directly related to perimenopause?' I thought, 'YES, yes, it is!' The shedding of the layers, layer after layer after layer. And really interesting that your hip is your trigger to the depths that you need to go to in order to peel back the layers.

So, let's look at one of those layers. How do you think those messages you received from your parents impacted on you as you transitioned from girl to woman?

I think I learned to be ashamed about being a woman, because it hadn't been seen or celebrated very often. There were little glimpses of time which seemed to match up with being an okay thing to be and do, and so that was great. But often my own authentic, wild self, did not match up with what was celebrated about being female or just being a child or growing into a woman. So, I felt this divide. In order for me to grow into the person I was meant to be, I had to leave my family. I had to move somewhere else. I could never talk about these things with my family, so it's not like I asked, 'Can I still be in a relationship with you and be myself?'

It didn't happen like that. But I felt like I needed to be away from all the people who knew me and my family and go somewhere where nobody knew me. And so, I did. And it was great! I loved it. So, that was a big impact.

Here's another thing that I only recently remembered in journaling about these things. Both of my grandmothers have died, one was dead before I was born. So I never met her, my father's mother. My mother's mother died when I was a teenager. I remember feeling worried that now that she was dead, her spirit might be able to see me and that she would be disappointed and disapprove of me. It's so funny, it just doesn't make logical sense, but it was a fear that I had. I could keep it together and hide from people if I could see them. It was my grandmothers mainly; I didn't worry about other dead people seeing me! It was her, the one that I had known, the one who I did have in my life up until her death.

Which I think is interesting. I really was concerned about keeping it together and showing the right side of myself to the right people. It was really hard for me to bring the parts of my two lives together, because I didn't know how to be, I didn't know how to act. I had relationships and boyfriends who would be like, 'What's going on?' when I brought them to meet my family, my parents. And they (boyfriends) would be like, 'What happened to you, where did you go?' This was the beginning of really starting to realise what was happening. It really wasn't a sustainable way to live – I couldn't keep everything separate all the time, compartmentalise everything and be healthy! So, that was a process.

I bought a house as a single woman; I was starting down the road of not following what my parents had wanted for me. I was a professional, I had my own car; I actually borrowed money from my parents to buy my first car and I paid it off in about half the amount of time, because I didn't like being in debt to them. I worked, I was fierce and ultra-responsible about being independent, because of that feeling that, in order to be myself, I have to be separate.

The hip surgery was another big, huge, thing because nobody knew I had the hip dysplasia until I was seventeen years old. Interestingly enough, when I was in utero, my mother learned about hip dysplasia because her friend's baby was in a brace, to help her hips develop in a healthy way. And she was carrying me in her womb and thinking to herself, 'I hope my baby doesn't have hip dysplasia.' And so, when I was born, she said to my paediatrician, "Check my baby's hips," and the paediatrician said my hips were fine, and my mother said, "Oh what a relief."

And then seventeen years later I was diagnosed with hip dysplasia during my college physical. I was getting ready to go far away to a new place where nobody knew me. It wasn't that far but it was *my* place. Luckily, all the doctors and the surgeons said they could wait a year, or until summer, until after my first year of college before they operated on my hip.

How was the surgery? What memories do you have of it?

The surgery was huge, I had just turned eighteen and the surgery was nine days later. So, in this time I was 'officially' an adult, in the way that I could sign my own consent papers for the medical procedures. And yet, I was completely unprepared for that role. Obviously, I had never done it before and here was this hugest thing, hugest medical decision of my life.

The procedure was very invasive. There was an orientation the day before the surgery. My parents and I stayed in a hotel and spent the day having the orientation at the hospital, where we met the anaesthesiologist and we learned about what was going to happen. We were shown a little video about what to expect.

I remember it clearly as there were two choices for me, either I was having complete anaesthesia and I would be completely unconscious during the surgery or I would have some kind of a spinal block, so that I wouldn't feel the surgery but I would be conscious during the surgery.

And I had just finished my first year of college and I had been reading for the first time in my life about feminism, and in particular the radical feminist's books and they had blown my mind! Completely. In particular one of the books by Mary Daly, called *Gyn/ecology*. I feel it would be interesting for me to read that again because I don't really remember anything about it. My 'takeaway' from it and what was influencing this part of my story, was that, she was talking about female genital mutilation happening in some cultures as a way of hurting women, and she talked about Chinese foot binding happening in some cultures, as another way of hurting women. And then she talked about Western medicine in a very similar way, especially in gynaecology. How science and medicine was going to save us from our 'troublesome' bodies.

So, I told the anaesthesiologist I didn't want to be unconscious during the surgery, I wanted to be conscious. I didn't want an -aesthesia, I think of Mary Daly – she does a lot of breaking down language, like re-membering, a-mazing. Anaesthesia is like the opposite of beauty, I can't remember exactly, but I specifically chose the spinal block. Then the next morning we were preparing for the surgery, and my parents said goodbye to me in the pre-op room. The nurses started my IV, they gave me Valium, so I was basically completely drunk. Then the anaesthesiologist came in and told me that I couldn't have the spinal block. Then the mask came over my face and I was put to sleep.

I was out for eight hours. And I feel like they stole something from me that I'm still trying to get back. I feel like it really disempowered me. And that I'm working really hard to get my power back. And as a perimenopausal woman it's become unbearable to carry this pain anymore, and to try and function in a disempowered state. I'm not going to do it anymore – and it feels so good to say that. I have a great therapist that I work with, and I have a body worker who I totally love. I had an appointment with her yesterday, which was amazing. I feel that, and she feels too, that my ship is starting in a new course – which feels really good, it's intentional.

Oh, my goodness Meg, that sounds powerful. How has that experience impacted on choices you went on to make?

That is really related to how these messages as a little girl and when I was turning eighteen, blended in with this other awful traumatic experience that I had. So, I wanted to mention the surgery, and I also wanted to say that luckily, and I'm *so* grateful for this – that I became a mother with midwives, at home. I was able to avoid the hospital, which was very intentional, and I'm so glad. I was intentional about planning home births because of my past experiences. And the midwives were huge in helping me feel good about my womb, feel good about my body and learn about what informed consent really means in medicine and in healing.

So, the disconnection from my authentic nature in terms of how I was supposed to behave and treat people and relationships is also how my body was supposed to also be denied of its true self.

The midwifery model of care is so different from the western medical model of care. For me it was like a big doorway into a whole other way of being that I just didn't know even existed. It raised the bar for me about what a healer can be. It's funny, their role is not to heal, their role is to catch your baby and take care of you. But they really helped me heal. I will feel forever grateful for my midwife and now I'm working for a school of midwifery because I feel so passionate about it.

I feel midwifery is so tied in with some of this wounding that women receive and midwifery is a healing gift. In the US, I think 10% of all births are tended by midwives and – that's crazy. I feel it's crazy how our culture just puts the female body up as being problematic and you have to be in a hospital where they're trained to treat problems. And so, then your body is just going to naturally be seen through that lens of 'this is problematic.'

And for the first time ever when I gave birth, I was the centre of my own care. I felt like I was important. Through my hip surgeries I did not feel that way. I was given the exact opposite message. So, to have my own body's wisdom honoured and encouraged was *huge*. My first birth – I almost didn't know what was happening. I was like, 'What do you mean I'm supposed to take responsibility for this process!' I had never seen that before. I had read about it, so I logically knew that this was how it was going to be. But my body on the other hand almost couldn't believe it. Like, 'What do you mean you're not going to tell me what to do and how to be and where to stand.' So, that was amazing. Then I was a mom – which is a whole other thing we can talk about.

I was shocked to find out my mother and father weren't the only people who thought motherhood should be part of that unfortunate programming, that a woman needed to be a mother in a certain way, within a certain parameter. Unfortunately, I was unprepared for that. But I think being a mother blew me open in a really wonderful way and I'm doing it differently than how society wants to have it done. And I'm really glad about that. And it's hard.

Your message here is so important to hear Meg. Thank you for sharing that power.

What memories do you have of your first bleed?

I was twelve and I knew what to expect, it wasn't a surprise to me. I think on some level I intuitively knew this process of menstruating belonged in the same category with all of the things we don't talk about and all of those inner wild yearnings that we might have, but we might not want to talk about. And also, at age ten or eleven, I was starting to see some of my friends become very slender and develop breasts and I was not seeing that in myself. I talked to my mum about that.

In particular, I had these knuckles that were dimpled, had these plump little pudgy hands. I remember some of my friends had knuckles that started to pop out. To me it looked more like a grown-up hand and I had a child hand. I talked to my mother about *that*, and she said that after I started my period, I would lose my 'baby fat.' So, the way I told my mother I had started my period, which was something I felt intuitively I should not speak about, was I just pointed to my knuckles!

I hoped she understood what I was trying to say. Eventually she figured out what I was trying to tell her. I had already helped myself to a box of pads in the bathroom. In fact, eventually I learned how to use a tampon reading the box instructions. My mother didn't help me out with any practical things. If I needed anything, I wrote it on the grocery list and she would buy it for me. So, no conversations really about any of that. The first bleed in particular, so I had pointed to my knuckles, and my mother said, "Oh, you're a woman now," and we went out for ice-cream, which was very nice but it still felt to me like we're not going to talk about this.

Did you want to talk about it?

No, because I didn't talk to my mother about things that I felt. I was told that I was very sensitive, like it was a bad thing, so I always felt like I couldn't. I could never show my sensitivity, or act like I didn't know what was going on. It would have been way too embarrassing to talk about with my mother. I think she might have felt the same way.

And where was your father in this? My mother taught me that it was absolutely forbidden to let my father and brothers see sanitary towels. I had to keep it all hidden.

I definitely was hiding everything. I'm sure my mother told my father that I had started my period – she might have even told him that in front of me. I didn't get the message that he wasn't allowed to know. I do remember one time, probably years later, that I was having menstrual cramps and my father filled up a hot water bottle for me. He's a very caring person. I didn't get the message that he would have been upset or embarrassed for me or whatever, but he and I didn't really talk about it that much. We didn't really talk to each other all that much anyway. He was at work all the time; he was busy.

So, you said at the beginning that you were prepared. You knew you were going to start bleeding; who did you learn that from?

That's a good question. I knew – I don't know how I knew! I know I had read books. There was young adult literature that I had read where I got some of my information about these things, about boys and relationships. I didn't get this from my mother, I got it from books and my friends. Probably the worst place to get it, like misinformation!

I remember trying to make my Barbies have sex with each other. I would pretend one of them was a boy – I had no clue. With the period, I knew blood was going to come out of me and I knew that was okay, that I was supposed to put a pad on my underwear. But honestly, I didn't know how often I was supposed to change the pad, it was a learning curve, and I was on my own, like it was basically trial and error.

We went on a vacation maybe six months later. We were gone for three weeks, and during that trip I got my period and I didn't know I was supposed to pack pads. I didn't know when it was going to come. It was a surprise every time. My mother might have packed them for me, but I know I was unprepared. I was sleeping in some borrowed sleeping bag at my relative's house, and I bled all over it in the night. I woke up my mother. I don't think I ever told anybody I got blood on the sleeping bag. I think I just hid it, but I needed a pad. I didn't know what to do, in the middle of the night. She had panty liners, she'd packed those, and she cut those apart and stuffed tissue in them and told me to use that. I have that memory and I always felt mad at my mum that she didn't pack very well, she was often unprepared, so I was unprepared. I have become a diligent packer! I hate the feeling of not being prepared.

Did you learn at some point to chart your cycle and if you did, who did you learn from?

I was very interested in it and I taught myself. I've researched and taught myself about it as an adult, because it fascinated me and I wanted to understand what was happening to my body. And I felt like I had to figure that out on my own, and so I did. And I was like the expert friend who all my other friends would ask about these things. And I did start charting it. I would mark it on the calendar because I felt it was empowering and also when I eventually started having sex, then I felt I was safer having sex knowing when I was going to be fertile.

When I first figured that out, I was so excited about it. And, what's an ovary?

What's happening? The bleeding part is the only part I'd ever seen, so that was the only part I'd had experience with. And the rest of it, I figured it out! Little by little. I thought it was fascinating – the fact that the energy I was feeling around ovulation was related to what my body was doing.... fascinating! I was around twenty-two to twenty-five years old.

I had a friend who was interested in women's health. She's now a healthcare practitioner, but back then we were waiting tables together. I went over to her house and she handed me a book Women's Bodies Women's Wisdom by Christiane Northrup. This was around 1995. I remember I loved that book. Every time I would go to her house I would want to look up and learn something new. Eventually I bought the book and it was my reference tool for what was going on with any part of my body. That was the first time I learnt about chakras. I was fascinated with the idea of the energy centres of the body and how they each give clues from the symptoms in the body about what's going on. I'm fascinated by our mind-body connection and the wisdom of the cycle and all of it. I thought it was amazing.

I was such a nerd, I kept track of it and I still track it. It doesn't happen regularly anymore, so I have this renewed interest in tracking it. My first skipped period I was convinced I was pregnant. It was the first time I felt I was having a 'scare,' an unwanted pregnancy. I took a pregnancy test and I wasn't pregnant, so I was like 'Oh, so what's going on?' Again, it was like going back to that feeling of, 'I don't know what's going on,' and this was perimenopause, where once again, after all these years, I'm back to not knowing. I feel I've been humbled. I don't know what's going to happen. I don't know when it's going to come and there's nothing wrong with that. It's just unsettling and uncomfortable.

Would you say the knowledge you learnt in that phase of your life has supported you now in perimenopause?

For sure, because at least I know what I don't know. At least I know I don't know something! I feel there are clues here to be discovered. I feel there's a richness and a depth to this, because I know I found this through other parts of my life, through my cycle, through my body, through my emotions and my energy. That paying attention to this now is like investigating, like a treasure map.

Did you know what to expect as you began your transition?

No, I still feel like I don't really know. My mother had hot flushes. I think I knew what that meant, that she was stopping her periods, but she didn't discuss it in detail. Every once in a while, she would take off her clothes and open up a window. One of the reasons I came to your group, Brier, is because I've been spending the past three or four years trying to find information. More than just information – inspiration and companionship on this journey because once again I feel like I have to be what I don't want to be. I feel like the culture wants me to be dealing with this privately and in secret on my own. And I don't want that for myself.

And actually, breastfeeding my baby was where I really realised for sure, that support from other women is amazing, it's gold. I went to a mother supporting mother organisation, after doing Tanya Dantus' Mother Empowerment Program, specifically for breastfeeding mothers who had forgotten how to breastfeed, because it's been stamped out of our mothering by the western medicine. So, that group of mothers supporting mothers through breastfeeding and also through all the different aspects of mothering was amazing for me huge, huge support.

And here's another aspect of my body that I don't understand, that I feel I need support for. Just a group of people, and books I've been reading (Susun S Weed). I found it to be wonderful! I knew I needed to find a group. I felt like I was grieving. I felt loss, and I wanted support.

I am so happy you found your way to my Menopause Wisdoms circle, Meg.

Second interview one year later

I am so excited to hear what is happening for you. Our last conversation was just so rich and a whole year ago! So, let's see how this flows and unfolds.

I'm excited too. I found my notes from last year and then looked at the prompts for what we'll cover today and I wondered if I would answer the questions from last year differently now.

Yes, that's such a great enquiry. I have wondered that too. I love the spaciousness that there has been between meeting and talking. I think that it's really perfect in relation to this transformational experience.

When I reflect on where I am at with the whole journey, being 'Baby Crone' feels like a good description of where I am because it's like I am learning. I have to learn a whole new way of being. It's still me and I still have memories of all the other ways of being that I have passed through.

The thing that I'm learning is that there is no predictability, there doesn't have to be. I don't have to be able to predict things. It's okay. In fact, I am starting to realise, and at first it felt like a negative that I could not predict. I didn't have the regular cycles in my body, but I feel like it's actually a gift. It's like a force, forcing me to feel free. Forcing me to be what I am, which is free rather than to put myself into constraints which I do – I do that.

It sounds to me like you are describing aspects of your initiation that you like.

Yeah.

Let's go with that flow then, is anything else emerging for you in terms of that.

Well, I think the feeling that in our culture growing old is seen as a negative and something to avoid. In some ways the fact that Menopause happens with age, it does feel like there is something to look forward to in a way. Like there is something new. If I'm in a rut, I can't be anymore because it's like this is fresh, it's like a new assignment, an opportunity. I can't be in a rut anymore, because Menopause is like a force, pushing me into a new way of being where I can't operate the same way I used to operate.

And that's good, I think if we didn't grow and change then we wouldn't feel alive.

I love the words that you used, the 'pushing through.' Menopause is a rebirth, we are giving birth to a new us, a new you, a new Meg. We push through and when we pass that point of resistance, just like in labour – the point where we are getting ready to push – we scream, "I don't want to do this anymore, this is too hard, this is too challenging, I don't like it," and then boom! There's no space for 'no.' Menopause is the time we need to be with that force of the new emerging and the opportunity that comes with that. That's why I think 'Baby Crone' is such a lovely turn of phrase.

Yeah. It's like I am new. I mean, somebody looking at me might not think I look new, but there are aspects of me that are brand new and unfamiliar and interesting. I am curious about it.

And sometimes I'm afraid of it too. I feel like there is a parallel between me and the way I really am and the natural pulls and pushes and connections, and then the culture that I am in, where these things aren't welcome or not recognised. So, the fact that those two things have to exist all in my one life, that is the problem. The problem is, not what is going on in my natural life inside of me and my psyche and my body; the problem is that I also have to be in the world.

And I have messages coming at me that are not natural, that are not helpful.

I'm sorry to hear that. Those negative attitudes from external situations are challenging. Are you feeling that with being this Baby Crone, with this wisdom that is coming through, the very natural, wild wise woman, are you feeling more adept and more equipped to deal with those challenges?

I think so, in some ways. I feel like I am looking at it from a different point of view in a way. It doesn't feel personal anymore. It doesn't feel like those messages are for me personally. I feel like I don't care as much about that, but I recognise it.

I still feel torn, you know. Should I participate in this or not? It's hard; it's hard to be the one not participating in what everybody else is just going along with and just doing it. It's lonely, it can be hard to find other people who understand that frame, that way of thinking or that way of being. And so personally, I think that's the biggest struggle, feeling like I am all alone.

I choose to homeschool my kids. I choose not to go to the doctor every time I am 'supposed' to go to the doctor. Those are just a couple of them. I have this longing for a spiritual community but I don't know where that exists the way I want it to. Because the faith that I grew up in with my parents isn't going to cut it. It's just not spiritually helpful for me. It's just the wrong messages for me. And it's not connecting to spirit in a way that's helpful for me.

I don't care as much about what other people are doing anymore. But

I do kind of look at them and I think, 'You all look like you are having fun together over there.' You know – doing the things like agreeing to just go along with things, dyeing your hair, straightening your hair, putting on tight clothes that look sexy and all the make-up and, you know, all that.

I hear that. I think it is interesting you say they look like they are having fun. But if we just peel off that first layer, they may well not be having fun but are actually caught in the patriarchal trap.

And they may be looking at you and sensing your freedom. When people who are not free, see or sense others who are free, there is a real edge to that.

We are the new witches, the new weavers and it can feel lonely, especially at the moment.

Because of the restrictions in response to Covid-19, we can't do the things that come naturally to us.

But we're not alone; there are many of us and more and more women, especially when we come to this point of Menopause, are having that realisation that this is the time to rise up and reclaim the true nature of ourselves.

Yeah, and learning to connect to what feels good in the body. I realised there are many different layers of that. There is the me thinking about it, but that can only do so much; me and my thinking mind. That's only one teeny tiny part of my body. And it's used to being in charge, you know. The culture that I was raised in is very puritan. I think it must be a tool of the patriarchy, this idea of being ashamed of natural bodies, of bodily function. Having to hide them and control them, it's been really hard. It's hard to not feel that creeping in.

I love my job because it's the opposite of me feeling lonely. When I'm doing my work, I'm with people who are like-minded, who seem to get it. Everybody is different. I'm definitely the oldest one working there and I feel that it can be kind of a fun role. But it's new for me to be the oldest person in a group.

At work I was reading about someone who identified as a full-service sex worker. This person wanted to become a midwife, to serve people in their community. And I was like, 'Wait, what?' I had that puritan feeling of like,

'What is this? A sex worker, who is open about what they did for work?' I actually had to look it up because I was like, 'What is a full-service sex worker?'

I didn't even know, and I was reading it and I was like, 'Is this okay? Isn't this illegal?' I had all these thoughts coming in. And then, you know, it's new, different; there's lots to learn all the time.

And the fact is, there are a ton of people who are full-service sex workers, who are not getting medical care. They have their own special medical needs, healthcare needs, especially in relation to their reproductive life. But that puritan voice inside of me, it was very strong asking, 'Does this person belong in an institution of education?'

It's so powerful and it's another gift of the Menopause, this process that you are going through, choosing the way that you are going through it. You are aware of those voices, those learnt beliefs and giving space to question them.

Yeah, I was asking, 'What is going on?' I never even thought about the rights and the justice for people working as full-service sex workers. And it's a great opportunity.

There are so many people in the world who never think twice about it. A privileged, upper-middle class white lady who is sitting in her little beautiful house with her little beautiful family – and I'm talking about myself – who has no awareness of what is really going on in many parts of the world. And even, probably, right in my own town.

It's a whole other element of reproductive justice. There is a drug that's not available in the United States, that can bring on uterine contractions. It's used in other parts of the world to end pregnancy. You can do it yourself. You can take the drug and it basically induces a miscarriage for an unwanted pregnancy. I didn't even know about it. I was reading about it at my job and my first thought was, 'Oh what a terrible thing to do, ending a pregnancy this way, all alone without the care of a practitioner.' And then I realized, there's that voice again! So being in a female body is political because the patriarchy wants to control what we can and cannot do with our own bodies and I have totally internalized all of those patriarchal rules. Not totally, I questioned them, at least I noticed.

It's so ingrained and is so part of my life experience that I feel like I couldn't even bring this up in conversation with most of the people I know. I think they would look at me like I'm crazy. These topics of conversation, people who would induce their own miscarriage, manage their own abortion or somebody who would openly admit to being a full-service sex worker, are just not discussed.

I feel Menopause is another one of those topics. People will talk about it but not as a positive transformation.

I've tried talking about it with people. Sometimes people will talk about how they are having cramps. And I think, 'Oh they still have their period.' I haven't had my period in many months now. I still have my cloth pads in the bathroom closet, I look at them sometimes and I feel kind of sad.

Because I might have it again, my blood might come back but I don't know. It's weird.

Yes, that not knowing is a very interesting space to be in.

Taking part in this book Meg, you are a pioneer in speaking about Menopause, getting it out there and sharing it and being curious. You will be planting seeds with those people that are still resistant to the alchemy.

Let's look at the sexuality question. You have spoken about your internalised attitudes and responses around sex in relation to your work. How do you feel about sex and your sexuality at this phase in your life?

It's so interesting. I don't have the same level of desire that I used to have and I am curious about that. I find myself not knowing how to articulate this but my husband is very sexual, I know that about him. We have been together for thirteen years now and it is one of the things I love about him. It is important to our relationship. I find that we are still a match but I find he usually is the initiator these days. And for me it is more about what I want that has changed, from the whole concept of just trying to have an orgasm. That is gone. I do have them but that isn't the driving force. I don't care about that much. Sometimes it's just not going to happen; I can just tell.

But with him, it's like I can be connected with him and I love that. It's like we are joining our two energies and it's not about talking to each other. It's about doing it with our bodies, like joining, coming together, which I feel I love. And so, I think it sort of makes sense – biologically my body isn't trying to make a baby anymore. Sex is different. About a year ago I was bleeding for forty days in a row and that was not sexy. This is different, a new phase of what is going on in my womb, learning to ask, 'What does my body want now?' And it doesn't feel constant at all; it comes and goes. It feels powerful. My desire, it's very slow to kindle, but once it kindles, it's much bigger and much more. It's powerful, very powerful. I know he feels that too, but yeah, it's elusive.

Is it something that you talk about together?

Yes, we talk about it.

About your changes and your desire?

Yes.

And has that been an easy thing to do?

Yeah, he's very easy for me to talk to. I talked about those two parallel realities. He's so into that. It seems easy for him to shut out all of the 'shoulds' of society and he's not ashamed of talking about things. He's male and I think the patriarchy has served him in ways that it has not served me. I mean there are still some ways he doesn't really get everything I talk about. But yeah, we talk about that for sure, the desire is different. And, it doesn't scare him or worry him. He's a very enthusiastic and welcoming and open kind of person, especially sexually. I think he definitely finds me sexy, which I love. He is not part of those outside voices at all. So, yeah, we do talk about those things.

That is so beautiful and such a lovely message.

For many women the desire has completely gone and they are happy with that. It's different for each of us and so important for us to know that it is different.

I hear and read a lot, the view that we can be sexual and enjoy sex as elders. And it is often said in such a way that if we don't want that, we can be fixed. So, hearing from women themselves the different experiences around sex is helpful. And everything that has gone before impacts on our entire menopausal journey, including our sexual relationships and experiences.

Totally. Yeah. I feel like having the memories of my past sexual attitudes that I have passed through in my life has become more present in a way. The memories of experiences I have had. I have only been with my current partner for 14 years. And I never really intended – it wasn't my plan or my dream or my goal to get married and have children. Before we met, I was having other relationships as an adult. And I am so glad I did because I can remember all of these different chapters of Meg. I am the only one who knows all the different experiences that I have had. And I really cherish them. I mean even the ones that were painful or, you know, obviously I didn't marry those other people. I didn't for some reason – it wasn't a fit, for a long-term relationship, but boy, the sexuality and learning and being intimate with different people has been a real gift. And I'm glad about that. I love thinking about the memories, it's just fun. It's like, 'Oh yeah, this is my current state,' which is interesting and curious, but the memories are, 'Oh wow! I really did those things. Wow!' It was fun at the time.

It's interesting, you bringing up memory, not necessarily about sexual, intimate relationships, but memories per se. I found as a menopausal woman and particularly as a post-menopausal woman, I have really odd, random specific memories, like being in the car at a particular roundabout in London. I find that intriguing.

Me too.

I wonder what that place, that moment, at a cellular level is reminding me of. I find that fascinating.

Yeah. I do too and that same thing happens to me too, like why am I thinking about that person, the man I lived with for five years? He rarely comes into my psyche, I don't dream about him, I don't think about him, I don't long for him, I don't remember what it was like to be intimate with him really, but there is a call to remember. It's interesting.

My brothers will talk about certain things from our childhood and I will be like, 'Yeah, I don't remember that.' I don't remember it at all. You're right, other random things like the road, the sidewalk I used to walk on where I lived for just one year of my life, I think about it a lot and this coffee shop I used to go to. That year was really a profound year for me.

Well, there you go. There will be gifts in those memories.

Okay, so how about we dive into your womb energy?

I have had an interesting relationship with my body. As I said earlier, I had a birth defect and I feel like the process of creating life inside my body really shifted something very profoundly for me. It showed me that I am really more than I give myself credit for on a physical level. I revere my body in a new way after having the experience of child birth twice. And I really feel like that is womb energy, that is magic, total magic. I really wish more people could experience natural labour and delivery. Because I know a lot of people don't ever have that. They never naturally go into labour. There are interventions.

That feeling of my womb deciding it has its own personality and its own mission. It was not anything to do with me. It was me, but not consciously. That feeling, I felt like I was being rushed on a train track. And it was scary and the midwives, the women who were with me, they changed my life by holding space for that. They kept me focused, looking at me and saying, "Yes, this is right. Yes, you are great, you are doing great," because this really is how it's supposed to be, like this feels scary. They see it every day, like, 'Oh wow! Like wow!' I have been in this body all these years and I have never experienced this before. But it was amazing and it was really empowering.

After my second birth I never returned to regular periods and I tracked it because I missed it. I wanted it back again, that was seven years ago. But I feel like I have to remember that memory and realise this is the same womb. It still has its same wisdom that it had in that moment pushing that baby out. It is apart from any decisions that I am making. And I have to learn to try, I have to be that midwife for myself, just like, 'Yes this is good, this is right.'

It feels a little weird but this is exactly like you said, it's everything unfolding and exactly as it should, which is hard to remember sometimes.

I love how you are talking about feeling and remembering that power of the womb and giving birth. Did you feel that connection at that time of having your babies? Or is this something that has come in for you now as a woman with the changes that your womb is undergoing?

I think it is coming to me now a little bit. I mean I feel like my relationship to my womb as a younger woman was very much trying to control it or trying to figure it out. In pregnancy I realized there was no way of controlling it. I have no control over this I am not actively creating this life inside of me. I cannot decide that it is going to go a certain way. Like oh my! Where is my placenta? I didn't decide to make my placenta go where it did and that was kind of a problem. Or maybe it could have been a problem and then it wasn't a problem but it was like, 'Oh yeah, I have to surrender to this.' And I realised, if I had learned that lesson earlier in my life, I would have enjoyed my body more. That whole controlling, patriarchal attitude was very present in my entire adult life. I learned it at puberty.

The gift of the Menopause for me was to unravel all of those learnt attitudes and behaviours. Not just for me but for all women present and past, our daughters and sisters and our mothers and grandmothers. It is time to change the narrative and heal the wounding. Time to tell 'herstory.'

It is time. Yeah, we need to start celebrating the wisdom of our body rather than feeling ashamed of it. I think I have made progress beyond where my mother was on that, which is great.

Well, let us go to your mum then. Your experience is different to how you observed your mother's to be. How old were you when she was going through her menopausal years? Did you know when she was going through it?

Yes, she was going through her Menopause the same time I was starting my menstrual cycle for the first time. I don't know if that is common or not, if our two bodies were talking to each other? She did say that when I started menstruating, she started getting her period again, when she had not had it for a while. I have had relationships with other women where we seem to be *in sync* that way. But she talked about her hot flushes and she would throw open all the windows and rip off her clothes.

One of the ways of communication that was in my childhood home was humour and sarcasm and it is something that I have stored in my adult life. I can be humorous but I try not to be rude or to tease or belittle as a way of being funny. But back then I was still trying to communicate with these people I lived with. That was how everybody talked to each other – we teased each other, you know.

I used to be rude to her about her hot flushes as a way of being funny and she thought it was funny and she laughed about it. She has told this story repeatedly ever since and laughed at how funny it was, that I said to her, "It's a good thing you are having hot flushes this summer or we would have nothing else to talk about."

When I think of that now I feel like I would *never* say that to someone ever. Now, that feels like cancelling out somebody's experience but she thought it was hilarious. It's her currency, this is how she is, you know. So, she loves telling that story. I think I don't really connect to the motivation I had for saying that to her. But I think it's strange that that has now become a family story that gets told.

We were the two females, I had brothers and a father, but we were the two, the only two female bodies in the house. I don't think she celebrated Menopause very much. I know she didn't take hormones which other people her age were doing. I think her doctor tried to get her to do it but she grew up on a farm and she understood about natural processes from the animals, and so she didn't think taking hormones was a good idea. She thought that was weird. She had her grey hair and white hair and so in that way it is good.

She always grappled with her weight. She wasn't overweight but she was always putting herself on diets and then she put me on diets. One time, she cut out this pink pig and put it on the refrigerator and it said, 'Do not pig out,' which was a sign for the two of us, but not for anybody else in the family. I liked corn on the cob a lot when I was young and she used to tell me, when I was enjoying a beautiful corn, she would say, "Corn is what they fatten pigs on," because she was a farmer and her father grew corn to fatten the pigs and that's probably what he said. I don't think she was intuitively connected with her body; I think she was very much listening to the messages from the beauty culture that it's not good to be overweight.

I feel like I have progressed to a different state of awareness. I have been trying to manage my thyroid condition with nutrition and I've changed the foods that I eat. As a result, I've lost weight and she's told me how good I look now that I've lost this weight. She knows that I'm doing this because I have a diagnosis. I've told her that but she still tells me, "Oh well, you look good."

I think the Menopause for her was a nuisance. There was no deeper connection, not that I'm aware of. She didn't talk about it.

Are you able to have this sort of conversation with your mum, would you want to?

No, not unless I could make a joke out of it. No, she shuts me down pretty quickly when I go deep. She just says things like, 'Oh don't be so sensitive,' like it's a bad thing.

I don't bring her into my innermost circle, I have grieved that. I have done a program in healing the Mother Wound because it's troubled me my whole life that my mother, my own mother, is not a force of grounding and nurturing the way I want her to be. Now that I am a mother, I know that no one person can be everything to anybody else. And so, I've grieved, I've been grieving that, feeling like somebody in my life should be able to help me navigate this time in my life. You Brier, you are helping me navigate this. But it's interesting how few people are connected to this phase of life as a gift.

It resonates so much with me what you were saying about your mother and healing the Mother Wound. Menopause has certainly helped me to continue to heal more layers of that wounding. Just recently I was able to let go of something and forgive my mum for not being or doing a thing that my inner child, my little girl had wanted her to be and do.

Yeah, and that is very empowering.

It is empowering, being able to recognise that I don't want to hold onto that piece anymore, because it doesn't serve me, is beautifully liberating. It allows me to step into my sovereignty.

It is time to grow up. It's like we can be our own force – we can be the force for our own selves that we were looking for in our mothers. And once I realised that, I was like, 'Oh she is just a person I have a relationship with.' I don't have to hang so many hopes and dreams and heavy stuff on her anymore. If there is something I need I can get it for myself because I am a grown-up now. I can grow up. She was doing the best she could and I love her, you know. And I am doing the best I can. Everybody is doing the best they can. It's very freeing to forgive other people for sure.

That is such a powerful example for us to model to our daughters. We can stop the wounding in our lineage. Connecting to our ancestors and being grateful for all that they did, all that they experienced, this is healing for our mothers too. And for us to now cut the cords which bind us to our wounding we can be grateful for all of the gifts that they brought and hold on to those.

I read last night a description of how within our life tapestries, there are certain threads that are being pulled so tightly, it distorts the story. But once we release it, it brings back balance. I thought that was such a beautiful analogy.

I felt I didn't need to pull on that thread anymore. I can free myself, and it then frees the other person.

I have been thinking about ancestors and my family line recently. I didn't know my grandmother, my dad's mom, because she had passed away before I was born. And I felt like that was a mystery I wanted to solve and figure out. I was asking myself, 'Who was that woman? What was she like?' My other grandmother, my mother's mother, I did know. I had a relationship with her but I wasn't that old when she died. I wasn't an adult yet. I remember feeling worried that now that she was in the spirit world that she would know things about me.

So, I love the idea of cutting that type of cord. I'm not tied to all of those 'shoulds' and all of those 'be a good girl' kind of messages that come from my family and that were handed down to me probably because of survival, but I don't need those anymore. I don't need those messages and I can cut the cord. I love that cutting, that cutting the cord and letting go of that string. Like nope, I don't need that anymore and I choose to imagine that my ancestors are with me in very positive nurturing ways and helping me and guiding me. And that they have also forgotten all of those unnecessary things, that it's not necessary anymore to think about that.

Oh, so beautiful and a perfect place to bring this to a close. I'm thinking Meg that perhaps we could have a cutting of the chord ceremony in the Menopause Wisdoms online Circle?

That's a good idea. That would great! And thank you Brier for writing the book. I cannot wait to see it. Thank you. Thank you so much.

It has been a pleasure. I have been really moved by your honesty and grace in sharing your story. Thank you, Meg.

Reflective Questions

What resonated with you from Meg's story?

What insights have you gleaned?

What is your biggest takeaway?

MIA

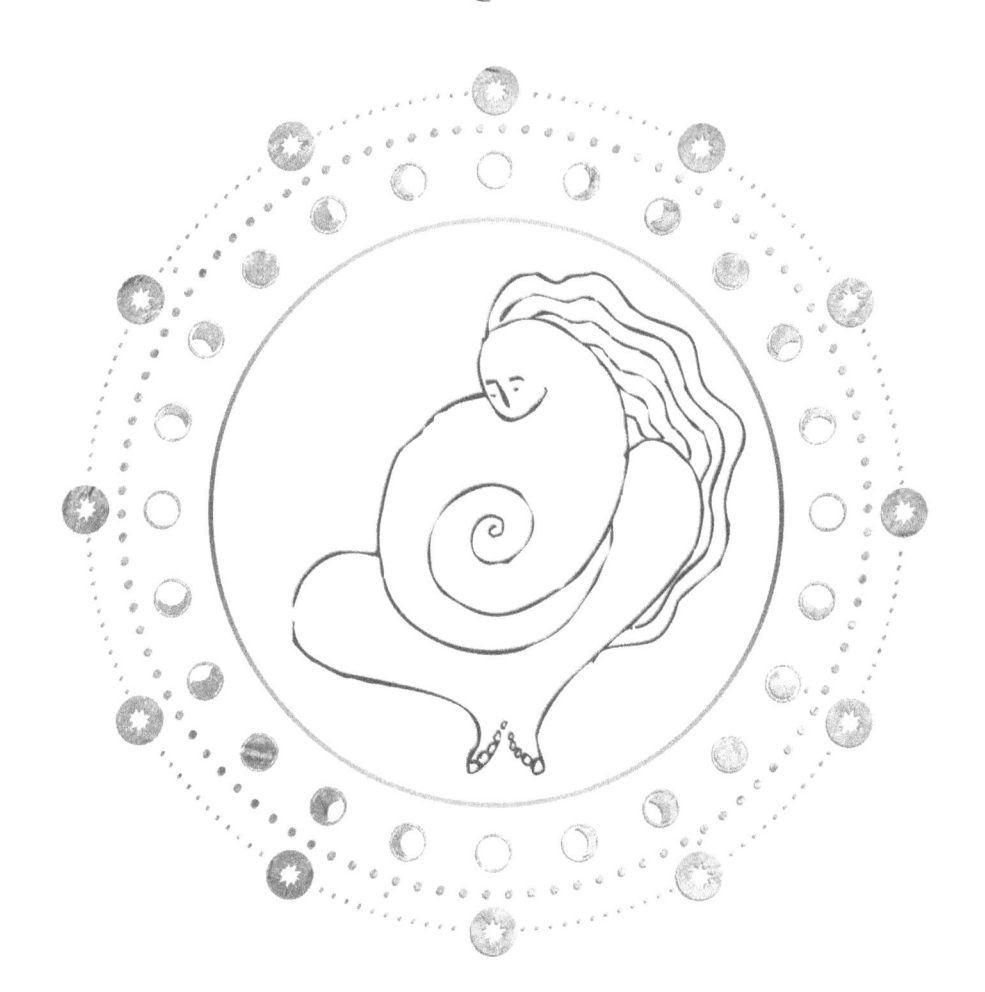

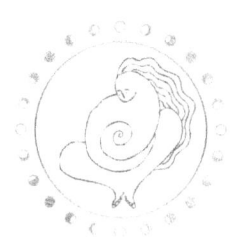

Thinking back to the first messages you were given from your mother, father, friends and media what were you told, taught and shown about what it is to be a woman?

There was very little information that was given to me around that, not directly. Obviously, it was all around me, women modelling in their own way, and there were always cultural images, but I don't feel like I grew up with a sense of what it's like to be a woman at all. Not consciously, it wasn't something I was thinking about consciously.

Did you see other women and think, 'I want to be like her, or look like her'?

No, I don't have any recollection of that. I haven't got an awful lot of memories of childhood or being a teenager. When I started bleeding, I felt like I'd been hit over the head. It felt like a very rude awakening into a reality, a change. That's what it was like for me. There must've been women that I saw that I thought I liked, but I don't have a conscious memory of it. It wasn't present at all, that awareness of what it's like to be a woman in the world. That came later on.

A lot of the things to do with the body, even like the practicalities of having a period and what to do when you're bleeding, stuff like that, I got that information through friends and a little bit through one of my aunties, who is just two years older than me, and we literally grew up together. She was quite free in her expression. So, if there was one person I would have looked at, it would've been her. To me she was just so free and doing naughty things, but I felt too inhibited to even discuss stuff.

Let's go back to what you said about feeling like you'd been hit over the head when you started bleeding. What had you been told, if anything, about what to expect?

Again, very little, the bare minimum. At school we vaguely had some sex education, but it was like, 'This will happen.' 'These are the organs,' and that was basically it. It wasn't very enticing and I always felt awkward about it, that was the main thing. It's always been awkward in my body, I haven't been much in my body. When I look back, at being fourteen, fifteen years old, I had scoliosis and on a purely physical level, I know that explains these feelings. I've got one leg shorter than the other. But later on when I started studying the energetic body, scoliosis is one of the giveaways of someone who is not in her body. Because it literally pulls the spine out of shape.

Did that impact on your cycle? Did you have pain. And did you have any awareness of being cyclical?

Yes, I was aware of my cycle as being very regular. But I remember cramps, and headaches and feeling like I didn't want to be around anyone else. But I wasn't aware of a sense of connection with it. It was something that was happening to me every month and it was pretty annoying! It was a hindrance, because I was so uncomfortable. I was uncomfortable in my body, going to school. It was like having that paranoia that everyone around me knew that I was bleeding. It was so obvious and I remember particularly being really sensitive about how I smelt, just being really awkward about being smelly and constantly having to wash because I felt really uncomfortable with the smell of it. So, it wasn't something I was enjoying at all, and not something I was connected with in other ways.

I was told it was The Curse. Did you ever hear it referred to as that?

In France, well not so much that. But I was aware of it being woven with Eve, the whole story around Eve and from then on, women had to endure. The basic Catholic upbringing. The whole thing was like something you had to endure.

And was that an attitude of your friends, would you say their experience was similar to your own, and did you talk about it with them?

Not much, no. I don't remember that. It just came up in conversation like, 'Let's go to the beach,' and saying 'No,' because I'm bleeding. Just things like that, coming up as another disadvantage. It was in the way. Later on, I remember there was a conversation around tampons. When they first came out and started to be more used, we shared stories on using tampons. There were those two methods, so we compared notes. It was either the practicalities or how it was a bore to endure that. It wasn't until later in my twenties when I started to go out in the world a bit more and meet different people and have different experiences. I then started to have different conversations.

So how do you feel those early experiences impacted on your views of what it is to be a woman? Did you suddenly shift your feelings of it being a pain, of being awkward, something to endure or do you think you carried that through?

I think I carried it through for a long time. Probably until, I say even to this day there are areas I'm still not comfortable with. If there's one area, I'm not totally comfortable with, it's my womb. When we started this conversation with your womb meditation, checking in with our womb and you spoke, "Just say hello to your womb."

I was like, 'Oh, hello!' I just don't go there! It's not a place at all, not consciously anyway, that's part of my routine.

How is not being connected to your womb impacting on you as a menopausal woman?

Well, I think the thing that brought me more in touch with my womb space and my body generally and my cycle was becoming a mum. That really opened up quite a lot of doors, in the sense that suddenly I was brought back into my body. From there I was a lot more present because being a mother I didn't want to be anywhere else. I wanted to be present with my child.

There was always a sense that I would be flourishing or flowering later on in life. I always considered being fifty as being something to get to. It kind of makes sense now. Being on that side of fifty, I feel a lot more comfortable within myself. There are still areas of discomfort but I'm a lot more comfortable, a lot more present and I'm enjoying using my body as a tool.

So, the way it has impacted on the Menopause and possibly on the early years when I started to have lots of distraction, was that instead of having curiosity about it, again I was falling back into, 'Oh that's something that's happening to me, and it's an inconvenience.' So, in the first years of Menopause, when I started to be more present with it, to explore and to feel into it, I would say that's more recent. The last couple of years really, since I have stopped bleeding.

That's interesting that it was the cessation of the blood that brought you to that place.

That definitely brought something in to me because I felt like I wasn't being dragged through that every month. At one point it wasn't there, so, phew!

So, what I hear is that since you stopped bleeding you have more of a connection to your body but still not to your womb?

No, I started to have more connection when I did my Shamanic training because during that time, I came across other cultures and especially North American where the Red Tent emerged from. That was in my early thirties and I decided to study, so I would consciously sit with it.

But then I got pregnant, which is interesting because since then, I became a lot more connected with the cycle and just being aware and paying attention. But *not* with the womb energy or the womb space. That's still something that's not part of me.

Moving into your menopausal years, had you been given any information about what that transition was likely to be, in terms of the physical, the emotional and the spiritual changes? Did you know what to expect becoming a menopausal woman?

Well, by that stage, by the time I started to be perimenopausal, I was in circles with women and my curiosity was switched on. I would ask questions, I would listen to others stories, I read books, I got information. So, when it was happening, when it started to be disruptive, it wasn't like a shock, or a surprise or anything. It was, 'Oh, alright, that's Menopause!'

I was a lot more with it. Having those women's circles all those years was such a support. And to me, the Menopause is, you get this mental opening, and you have that space, it's just *so* precious. I mean, 'Oh my goodness me.'

And I'm so thrilled that culture of conscious cycling and being aware is emerging. All these young women who are doing that from their twenties or from the first time they bleed – all that wisdom, every month for thirty years.

Wow, yes, that's potent, isn't it?

Yes! It just feels so strong in the world. In some ways I just have to grieve that I didn't follow that path, but I am so grateful to have had that support during those stages where literally the floor was going from under my feet. It felt like it anyway!

Can you recall your mothers experience of her menopausal years? I'm guessing she wasn't sitting in Circle with other women? Did her changes happen when you were still living at home?

No, I'd gone by then but I was still quite close. I moved away when I was thirty-one and I think my mum had just finished bleeding by then and she was going through Menopause. It was really interesting, I had this conversation with my sister and with my mum being present. Both me and my sister have a memory of her going through the Menopause and she is in total denial about it. She says she remembers having hot flashes but not feeling like it was a terrible inconvenience. She remembers it as sailing through it perfectly. Whereas me and my sister remember how much she hated herself, the mood swings. My mum has always been a bit of a hypochondriac, but during those years it was just like, 'Wow, okay!' She was going out of proportions, swinging from one mood to another. There was obviously a lot of things she would supress. She got quite ill – the prognosis was to have her womb removed. At the time I had started to see a guy who was practising Chinese Medicine and I suggested my mum see him first before her hospital appointment and then take it from there. And bless her, she did and she didn't go to the hospital and have everything removed. I guess from the doctors perspective it was the classic 'hysterical woman.'

Yes, that happened to my mother.

Yes, so she was just not knowing what to do with what she was experiencing. She carried on seeing the Chinese Medicine doctor for a few years.

That's really moving. Had you not had your own wisdom around that to suggest an alternative to her, she would have had her womb removed.

Yes, and it wasn't necessary.

No, and they often weren't. And I know you've heard me say before, things have barely changed. When I went to the hospital about my uterine fibroid, the first thing I was offered was a hysterectomy.

I think because the medical profession has been educated that way, I suppose doctors expect or assume that we (women) just want it (our womb) taken away. You go to see the doctor and say, "I've got something wrong." That's the culture.

The interesting thing I found though was when they are confronted with someone who says, 'Actually I've entered onto a path of self-healing and I no longer have the symptoms that originally brought me here to get a diagnosis and no thank you I don't want a hysterectomy,' they don't actually hear that. So, when they're presented with something outside of that narrow box of, 'Please fix me,' they don't listen. They don't know what to do.

No, because then they have the fear of litigation. If they don't fix you and then later on you break down again you might turn to them and say, 'You didn't do your job.'

Yeah, I guess there's that, but I also think there's a strong element of they think they know what's better for you – they are the authority.

Oh god yeah! Especially if you're a woman.

And especially with something about your womb.

So, I know how supportive it is sitting in Circle with other women in relation to Menopause. It opens up pathways of healing. Even having had that, I still want to ask, are there any aspects you have disliked?

Yes, the physical upheaval. I would regularly get that feeling of my body shutting down, and that's probably something to do with adrenal fatigue. I looked into that recently because of something to do with my mum, I was reading all the symptoms and I thought, 'Oh! okay, that could explain everything.' What I was experiencing was strong headaches, strong nausea, my body completely shutting down. It would usually last two to three days, and all I could do was sleep. I had no appetite what so ever. Then it would stop, but it was happening regularly.

Was this linked to the Menopause?

Well, it was happening all the time during those years. How I understand it now is on the physical level, it was adrenal fatigue. On the energetic level it was showing me how much energy I was releasing. Having my adrenals in a constant state of stress and being menopausal, there was not enough energy there. My body was saying, 'Okay, shut down!'

So, I don't know if it was the Menopause doing it or if it was highlighted in that way. I get a sense that it was there. I saw it as an inconvenience, it's the Menopause. I'm starting to see it now as the Menopause actually teaching me something really important.

I love that switch in your perception. What about other symptoms, did you have hot flushes, insomnia, rage?

I think it was the rage first, coming out of the blue. One minute I was fine and the next minute I was out there with an axe chopping people's heads off! That sudden impulse of, 'That's it, I'm going,' that feeling of 'I can't be here, I can't do that anymore. I've got to be alone.' It was so visceral, that was the thing that really puzzled me, just how strong. Those were in the first few years.

The hot flushes, I still get them but I've been okay with it. I don't get the ones where you have to literally change the bedding in the middle of the night. They can get quite strong. I do get to the point of being quite sweaty but not drenching. I'm actually enjoying the hot flushes. Yeah, I like those.

Mmm, yes, I get that. I have found with my hot flushes, when they first started, they were very different to how I am experiencing them now. To begin with it was like a Kundalini experience, my body was vibrating all the way from my feet, up and out. Then it started in different places in my body and the heat came. And in more recent months the sweating, like you, not drenching, but really like, 'Fucking hell!' I literally have to strip off layers of clothing I get so hot.

Yes, I do that too.

So, the times I didn't enjoy, were being borderline suicidal, lots of times when I thought, 'What's the fucking point?' 'Why would I even want to have another day?' That was quite strong, that went on for a long time. I remember some days just being like borderline, always having to reflect on things when I'm in a pit. I'd grab the phone and talk with someone and cry. That was so valuable to have someone there. Sometimes it would make me feel better, but it was knowing that someone was holding my hand, I wasn't doing it on my own. And I have been thinking of younger women in their early 40s and starting to feel this and wanting to say to them, "Make sure you make some space to rest and don't do it on your own."

Be prepared as much as possible. We never know what the experience is going to be like, but you can prepare by knowing that there will be days when you can't function at all because you don't recognise anything. You don't know who you are anymore, trying to function normally and you don't know how to deal with it.

Although we are beginning to talk about Menopause, our own experience of being in Circle and being held by other women within a safe, loving space, it is still relatively rare. I don't think in general women are accessing that. So, for some women when they feel like what you describe here, they will automatically think they need to go down the HRT or anti-depressant route because alternative options are still not commonplace.

When we aren't given a different perspective to that of mainstream medicine, we continue doing all the things we usually do, ignoring our body's innate wisdom to want to rest, to reflect, to go inwards. There are still challenges and difficulties in dealing with the changes but with support and the knowledge that the Menopause is an alchemical rebirth, it can also be a phenomenal experience!

When we're conscious of the things that are happening, of how we can be with those things, explore them, move through them. We can then emerge the other side as a potent, powerful woman.

Yes, and that's the piece that really needs to be said more. And too, when women become a Crone, well, I think, and I know for myself that there is the bit between the Menopause and the Crone, that needs to be addressed too. Crone comes a lot later, and I think that the place that I am now is the one that the world really, really needs right now. Anyone who is behind the patriarch will be pissing themselves with fright, because Menopause is women in their whole power! You know, we've done the Motherhood, we've got experience. One of the things I absolutely treasure from Menopause at the beginning, I can still remember the day when it was like a switch being turned off, 'I'm not going to put up with that shit anymore.' It was such a moment, it was a realisation, 'Oh wow!'

So probably something is switched off and something else is switched on.

I love hearing you say that Mia. I had a similar experience which came out when I was writing my first book. It was a moment that gave me the title of the book. For me, it was a moment of realisation that I no longer had to have armour on, I no longer had to be the warrior in fight mode. Now I feel like I have a 'soft' power, I can still access my fierceness if I need to and I'm strong. But it's having an ability to speak my Truth from a place without the armour, from an expansive place, from a place where I can breathe.

I like that. It's like the breathing, doing something that is self-care. I was doing it because I had to, I didn't have any other choice. So, I hope these messages are going to reach younger women so that they know the more they are in touch with their cycle and self-care they can generate, the better it will be for themselves. And having Circles of friends, moving through life together and sharing. That's the message. Yay!

Second interview one year later

So, I wonder what new things have emerged for you with the space of over a year since we last spoke? The first question that we come to now is, how do you feel when you look in the mirror, if you do?

Well, my vision being what it is at the moment, I don't have my glasses – then it's quite convenient. And yeah, I really notice if I happen to be in front of the mirror and I've got my glasses, then I just notice the lines. It's not quite rejection but there is a sense of, 'Oh wow! Look at me, I am old.' There is a sense of turning away from that image.

It's difficult at the moment, this is something that's hot in the cauldron. Seeing my face in the mirror sends me right back to how difficult it still is to properly look after myself.

I need to really honour my body. So, I mean it's a lot better than it used to be but when I look at my face in the mirror and I see the lines and the colour and stuff, I can tell that I have not hydrated myself properly. That's what I see in the mirror, that's what it's telling me and that's what I turn away from, more than what I actually look like. I'm not that fussed about that but it really reflects back those years of not looking after myself.

That's really powerful to hear what you're having reflected back at you.

Another question that came into my mind as you were saying that was, do you ever look at your complete body, your entire body?

I do. When I have a bath or something, I look at my body. I'm more comfortable with it now. There is anger that I could have done it differently and probably my body would look different. But as you go through life, there's a lot that you can get away with when you're in your twenties and thirties, even your forties. And then you reach fifties. And so now I am just looking and it's okay. I'm okay with it, I'm slowly reconciling myself with what shape my body is now and the fact that I made it. I'm starting to move away from already being an old woman, you know, like older than I actually am.

I realised I wanted to be old prematurely. It's like I was already in the mindset of being an old woman and I had to acknowledge her and say, 'Well, I will see you later.'

It's like, yeah okay I am aging and the body is the result of neglects through the years but I want to encourage the juices that are still there as opposed to just going to that mindset of, 'Oh that's it.'

And I'm feeling, just acknowledging that is quite strong in response to the message that society projects onto aging women. I can see that it's changing but it's still present. I have been surprised sometimes, just out of curiosity, checking with women how old they are and seeing women that I thought were a lot older and actually they might be my age and that's because they have already gone into that mindset. Into being 85 years old, in the distance, way over there!

This is something I have been reflecting on recently. I'm going to be sixty in a couple of weeks and I have lots of thought processes going on around what does that mean and how many more years have I got left and how different will it feel? If the next ten years go as quickly as the last ten years, I am going to be seventy in a nanosecond. I find it really fascinating to think about that, how differently time seems to move now I am older.

Well, I am lucky in the sense that my grandmother is still alive. She is going to be ninety-seven next month.

I'm still having conversations with her. I'm lucky because I can look at her and say, 'Yeah that's me in forty years.' And it allows me to go back to that place of being the grandchild, the granddaughter with my grandmother. I really appreciate that.

It's good to have older people in your family. I remember when my dad's mother died, I was there in the room and my dad turned around to me and said, "Well, that's it, I am next."

His parents were gone, his older brother was gone, so, you know, chronologically, yes, he could be next.

I feel lucky that I still have my parents and my grandmother. And I know that it doesn't really mean anything but I feel like it's almost keeping death away from me for a little bit longer.

I can sense how that must feel comforting. My grandparents all died when I was a small child and as a young adult, both my parents are dead too, so I don't have access to that thread of thinking, but I like it!

Okay, so the next question.

What are your feelings about your sexuality and sex as a menopausal, post-menopausal woman?

Well, that is still completely out of the picture.

And how do you feel about it?

I don't miss it. I'm aware that I'm probably missing out on something though, if that makes sense? It's kind of always on the periphery. I mean I'm really appreciating the Menopause journey over the last year. I think the circumstances (Covid 19) are awakening the world. It's been working for me as well. I've really appreciated the journey and there were times during 2020 where I had glimpses of possibility, of going back to being sexual. They were quick flashes but it felt like, 'Okay so that door is not closed, locked away.' My sense is that I will go back to it but I'm taking a long way around and there's other things that need to be integrated before I go back to it.

It really feels like at the time when I was a teenager and early adulthood when I became sexual, I didn't have a clue what it was, what sex was about. It was just something that you do because you are an adult. There was no sacredness in it, no thought about how it *could* be. It's just something that happens.

Is that the piece that you feel you are missing out on?

Yeah. I'm not saying that everything I'm doing is heading that way, but it feels, because we are having this conversation now, I'm trying to put the bits together. I'm taking a long way around but it might be at some point I will have to revisit that. Maybe what I'm doing and the pieces that I'm reclaiming at the moment. It's happening this way because it's heading that way, if that makes sense?

Yes, it does. If I remember correctly, last time we spoke you were doing some sort of work with another woman around sexuality.

Yeah. But I didn't go very far with it. It was like one of those times where I had a glimpse and I tried to go into it but I stepped away from it because it was just, 'Yes that's still on the shelf.'

I have noticed for myself as a post-menopausal woman that I prefer working through my challenges on my own, now I'm at ease with working through the pieces that call for my attention. In my own way, in my own time, rather than seeking and looking for somebody else to hold me in a container to do it. So, I'm really interested to hear you say that. Is that something that you're also feeling generally as a post-menopausal woman?

Yeah, that's probably the biggest piece I have worked with very recently – how much I was relying on an external view of who I am; just to constantly judge myself against other people and constantly looking for approval. It's very fresh actually, I did a Mysterium (deep retreat) this weekend and there was that moment of total revelation where I could see that shell, that skin next to me and I knew there was no way I could crawl back into it, although I wanted to. There is no way I can go back into it. So that's a really fresh awareness.

I can tell that my communication comes from a different place, that feels really good. I feel more solid within myself and not asking others, "Is that what you want from me? Is that what you want to hear?"

And I know the price of not needing that approval. The price of maybe being rejected or being opposed but I am feeling strong in myself and that is the piece that I have been calling. When they started with the vaccine, the anxiety arrived with my decision (to not have it) which is like, 'Wow, what is it going to be like for people who don't remember that thing of making your own choices in this climate? Because the marketing is just so tremendous.' And the expectation that we are going to partake is so monumental. I don't know what it's going to be like, so that really brought me face to face with that fear of confrontation.

And so, after that Mysterium weekend and really seeing that shell next to me and knowing I am not going back there, then I can talk about it and I can feel that it is okay. I don't have to agree with everything that everybody else agrees with. I can have my own voice.

I remember years ago, at one point during the Menopause, there was that moment of, suddenly I really felt something falling off me and it was like, 'Oh I don't give a shit what people think about me,' but that was more about how I looked or something like that. What I express is not just how I look or how I will appear to others.

So, you've started to answer the question then about how you feel being a post-menopausal woman. Is there anything else that you want to add?

Well, there is. My sister's eldest daughter just announced that she is having a baby. And that is the next generation. It was quite a sweet moment talking with her and with my sister about it. My sister was talking about her memory of when I told her that I was pregnant and it was like that moment of looking back in that corridor and knowing that those days for me are gone and maybe already sensing that I was the elder, the distant eighty-five-year-old. But before the eighty-five-year-old, there is going to be another one that maybe we can call the elder having that place within the family and within the community. The older woman who's been on a journey and has a voice. I'm not there yet but I am aware of that presence that is growing and settling.

Yeah lovely! 'Growing and settling,' I like that Mia, beautiful!

Yeah, the growing and settling is a conversation I've had with other women who are menopausal or just about post-menopausal. It's like between being menopausal and being an elder or an older woman. I think I have seen women trying to jump too quickly from one to the other. And there is that space in between where it's very juicy. There is an extra layer of maturing there.

Reclaiming, preparing the house to step into.

Yes, absolutely. It's something that's been in my head quite a lot, thinking about the Menopause journey in relation to when I became a mother. It's so similar in the process, isn't it? We go through the gestation period, then the labour and there's that point where you say, "No, I can't do this, I don't want to do this."

And then the birth and there's the baby. Suddenly you are a mother, and you don't suddenly become a woman who knows everything about being a mother. So, to me it feels very similar. My experience of becoming a mother was that there was an expectation that once you have your baby, you get on with it, you just do it. There isn't a container in which we are being held by the elders, by the women who are experienced, who have been mothers and are now Crone. I think there is a similarity of early motherhood to being a newly post-menopausal woman. Susan S Weed refers to it as being a 'Baby Crone,' which I like because you've got the baby and the Crone there together. It's a rebirth and you don't suddenly become that elder. As you say, there is the growing and the settling, I like that.

Wow!

Okay. So, the final question then is do you now feel connected to your womb and yoni energy?

Now yeah. It probably goes hand in hand with the sexual piece because it's not just having sexual relationships; it's like the whole creativity piece.

I'm more concerned with the idea to maybe find that space to be a lot more grounded in my body. I was reading a book recently and it's about a guy who was an Indian master. He helped a woman who was post-menopausal to start her period again in order to have a baby.

Wow!

I was reading that and I thought, well good for her, that's what she really wanted. But that got me thinking, you know, given the opportunity, would I go back to menstruating? And I'm clear that I am quite happy where I am! I'm becoming more excited about the years ahead. I'm just so lucky now, you know. I've got circles of strong sisterhood and this is just so lovely, so nourishing, so helpful to have that. I so wish I had that when I was a teenager and a young woman, but it just wasn't present and it just wasn't my story, but I have got it now.

And being in that place of having collected all these stories and all this awareness and having younger women coming and turning towards us and asking questions about what to expect. I'm looking forward to this and being able to tell them from a place of honouring that it just feels really good.

That's a perfect way to end, honouring and being in a place of it being and feeling so good. Amazing, thank you Mia.

You're welcome.

Mia sent me the following after having read her story before going to print. Her words are so powerful and clear, perfect for her closing comment.

We've inherited lots of beliefs about what it's like to be a woman, what's acceptable, what's 'normal,' beliefs around pain, around 'it has to be hard and difficult,' the Eve story and its consequences. It makes me feel that having the focus on the 'symptoms' of Menopause takes us away from the transformation and healing that is occurring during those years. Those symptoms to me are due to unresolved and suppressed feelings, including the ones passed down genetically, and I'm talking trauma here, not just physical disposition. It's like debris coming to the surface to be sorted out, what to reclaim, what to compost, what to recycle, what to discard.

Reflective Questions

What resonated with you from Mia's story?

What insights have you gleaned?

What is your biggest takeaway?

NICOLA

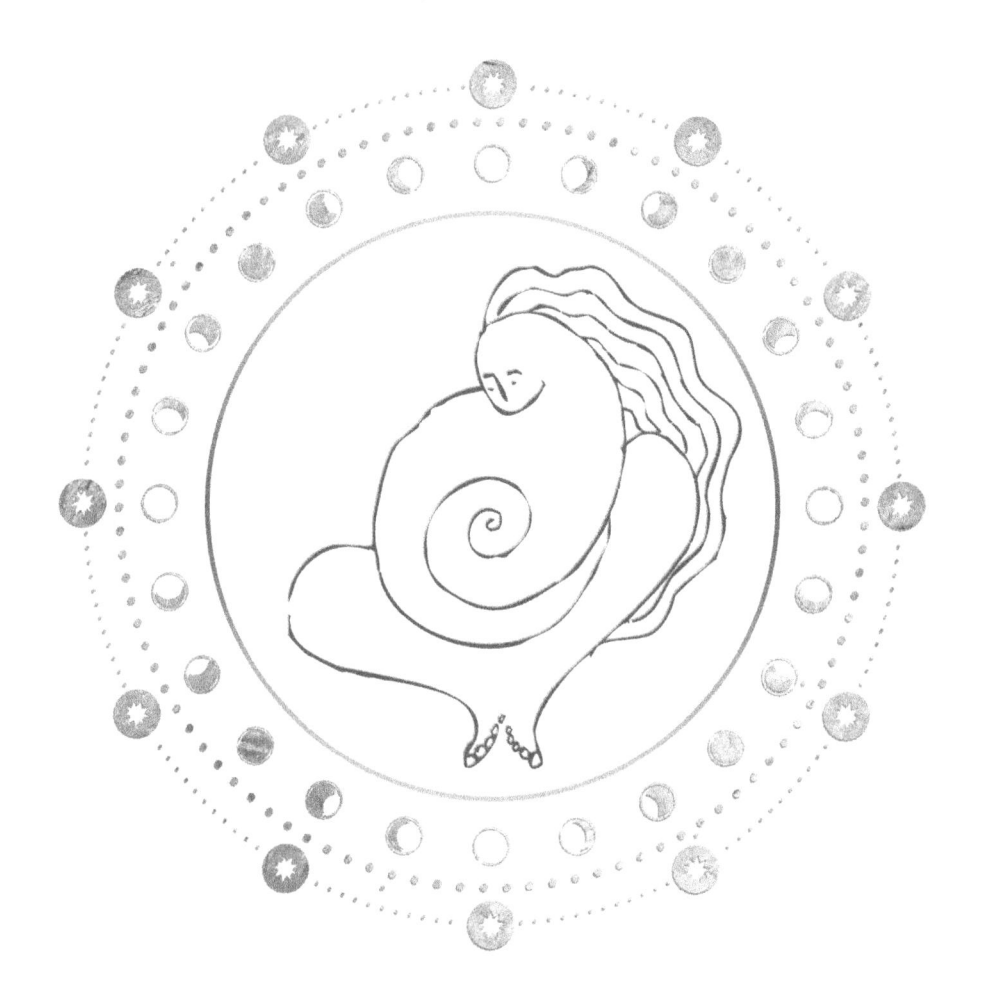

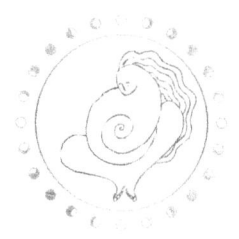

Where do you feel you are on your Menopausal journey?

It's interesting, I feel for the last year or just over a year, I've been experiencing symptoms of the Menopause. And it's interesting that I use the word 'symptoms' like it's a medical condition that needs to be treated, but I've been aware of the differences and changes just over the last fifteen months or so. So it feels, in some ways, I'm early on in the journey. But it's a journey really that I have no sense of how long it's going to last.

What have you been told or taught about what it is to be a woman?

I don't feel I was consciously told or taught anything about being a woman. I picked up everything unconsciously and most of that has been negative and restrictive. My parents were very young. They had me when they were twenty, so my mum was very young, relatively young, and she was an only child. My dad had two younger brothers and they were almost like younger brothers to me, so I spent a lot of time with men really, younger men.

They were the people who stood out in the family. And then when I went to University, I ended up living in a house with other guys – that was what I preferred. I lived in a house for at least a year, with three friends who were all men. I've always spent a lot of time, always been attracted for a lot of my life, to spending a lot of my time with men.

And I think the message I received about being a woman was that there's an inconvenience to it – the emotional bit. I remember when I was little, I can't really remember my mum displaying much emotion. I've spoken to her about that since. I think she really struggled quite often at times in those early years – well probably right through – she does still struggle to be honest. She likes to remove herself from a situation if emotions are coming up and that's something I've taken on.

She told me – I can't remember this happening – that when we were younger, she would just go off on her own in the car sometimes and just get away. My dad's mother, my grandmother on my dad's side, she was only forty when I was born. I saw her as an old woman though! I remember with her as well, every Sunday, we went over to my grandad and grandma's house for Sunday lunch, and my gran would always be in the kitchen, usually crying. I imagine she was going through Menopause, but it wasn't something that was spoken about. My grandad was an alcoholic, so there was a huge amount of tension in the family. It doesn't feel to me like she was supported through that. It was like, 'Gran's crying again,' or, 'Mum's crying again,' and it was just dismissed. As I said, it was an inconvenience, it was inconveniencing everyone else. And I think that was a message I took on, and actually even thinking back to me and my sister when we were little, my dad used to work shifts and he would quite often work the night shift, so we had to be quiet. I picked up the message to be quiet. I don't know if that was particularly gender specific, but they were messages that I picked up of how to be in the world.

When I look back, I think it was the messages from family that were the strongest, not so much media back then – I wasn't so aware of that. I think young girls now are so much more aware of it. But those family messages were very, very strong. And they came through from the female family members of my family and also the male members of my family. There was no discussion of what it means to be a woman, I can't remember ever any discussion around that. Or the different rites of passage you go through – nothing. It was just a non-issue, there was a lot of ignoring things.

Those are such powerful messages to be given, aren't they?

Yeah, it was all just shut down. And that wasn't the only aspect of life, virtually every aspect was shut down. Nothing was spoken about, it was all just, you just get on with it. My dad was very often grumpy and irritable, but he was more comfortable showing emotion than my mother. He would be the one to comfort us if my sister or I were upset. I remember my dad taking on that role. Or if there'd been arguments he'd always be the one to make the peace. My mum would just remove herself and not be the one to step in and make it okay and to soothe. So, I saw my dad being more in that role, which is interesting. I think that's something I've tended to take on from my mum. If there's conflict, I'll just remove myself and I'm quite happy if those conflicts are not resolved. I'll just be like, 'Okay, I can be with this.' That's changed now a lot through my relationship with my husband, but I wouldn't be the one naturally to step in and make the peace. I'll just remove myself.

How did those messages impact on you as you transitioned from girl to woman?

As I look back, I really have very little recollection of that time in relation to that transition. I remember that time in my life, but not in relation to making that transition from girl to woman. It feels like it was very practical, going through puberty, it was all handled in a very practical way, like going to buy my first bras and those kinds of things. Apart from that, nothing was spoken about. So, I didn't even think about it as a transition, it was just, this is what it is. There was no consciousness around it. That makes me feel sad.

Do you remember the day you had your first bleed?

Yeah, I do. I've got a very strong memory in my mind, it's very interesting. I can't actually remember the moment, when I knew I was having my first bleed or seeing the first blood. I can't remember that. All I remember is I must have told my mum; she'd already made sure that I had sanitary towels. I can't even remember how old I was, I must have been about fourteen. So, I had sanitary towels, she'd literally given them to me at some point, saying, "When you need them, here they are."

But no discussion around that, it was just, 'Here you go.' It was something to be avoided and absolutely not spoken about.

I must have said my bleed had come. I remember being sat in my room at my desk, I was doing homework and she came up to see me. The only thing I remember her saying to me is, "You should make sure you keep yourself clean. You should have a bath or a shower."

I think she also said something about making sure I ate plenty of fruit and veg, that was literally it. There was no sense of it being this important occasion or of it being honoured. That didn't even enter my mind, the idea that it could be. That perspective didn't come till way, way, way later, like fairly recently in my life. So, that's all I remember. And it was very brief. I don't even think it was my mum feeling uncomfortable, I just think it wasn't a thing for her either. She hadn't been taught or shown anything different to that. It was just this matter-of-factness and this is it, just look after yourself, keep clean – just very, very practical.

Was she secretive about her own menstrual cycle? Were you aware when she had her own bleed? Did you see her sanitary towels?

I remember seeing her box of Tampax in the bathroom but I can't remember it ever being spoken about it, even before I had my first period. The only time I remember talking to her about it was the first time I experienced period pain, and I thought I was dying. I don't know if it was the only time or because it was a new experience for me, but it felt so painful and I didn't know what it was. But I remember lying on her bed and I said, "Mum I'm going to have to go to the hospital."

And she was like, "No, you're fine." And that's the only other time I can remember us speaking about menstruation, either hers or mine.

Did you have that pain every month? Can you recall what your cycle was like?

I was pretty fortunate. I didn't really monitor it or pay much attention. It was pretty regular, I used to get a little bit of discomfort but I didn't really get anything that was debilitating. Again, I just saw it each month as a bit of an inconvenience and would carry on as normal, as much as I could.

And what about with your friends and peers? Your girlfriends, boys, was there any sort of teasing?

I can't remember with my friends really talking about periods. I think maybe I've just switched off from it because I really can't remember any conversations about anything like that. I do remember boys relentlessly teasing the girls about that kind of thing, about us smelling, the smell, I remember that. And just feeling, 'Oh my goodness.' I wasn't consciously thinking this, but I just picked up the idea that there was kind of something disgusting about being a woman. Like once I'd made that transition from girl to young woman that's when it seemed the boys would say horrible things. One boy in particular would go on about there's something different about us and there's something dirty and disgusting about us – that's the message I picked up.

So, how do you think those experiences have shaped your life as a woman?

Really, Brier, for most of my life, probably up until my late thirties, I wouldn't have even thought about what it means to be a woman, or my life as a woman. It just wasn't something that I considered or reflected on. I was always attracted to spending more time with men, obviously I've got my sister and we're very close, but even that relationship, it wasn't something we spoke about and actually I remember when I got my first period, she found my sanitary towels and she was going 'eergh' and teasing me about it, that kind of jokey, banter, all of that stuff, that's how my life continued.

It started when I was young with my dad and my uncles and then throughout school, University and into my work life – there was just that jokey detachment from life really, certainly from being a woman. I can't believe that now because I feel so different and it's happened in a relatively short amount of time. The only way I thought about being a woman was in terms of looking attractive and how could I look more attractive to men, basically.

Everything was just, God, I think I'm seeing it in quite a contrasted way, I'm probably being quite harsh on my younger self because there was a lot going on. I was shut down, I made decisions that didn't support or express who I truly was. You know, it was all very, very surface level – what looks good, not that that was consciously going on – but what looks good in terms of the decisions I was making, how I presented myself as a woman. It was all about looking attractive or acceptable. I used to work in a firm of financial advisors. I trained to become a financial advisor, I was the first woman to do that in this company. It was all guys, and I remember my boss, we used to go out for lunches, it was quite a sociable thing. At the time I was dying my hair, straightening my hair, and he said, "I'm going to take you out for lunch tomorrow, make sure you straighten your hair."

And at the time I just laughed or giggled or something, I mean obviously it registered because I'm remembering it now. It was all that, 'Look nice, tone yourself down,' and that's how my life was.

I speak to my husband about it now. Sometimes he's talking about women at work, it came into conversation recently, he doesn't see the difference. He sees everyone as equal. But I say to him that's not the experience people have. That's not the experience that I've had and I know it's hard to believe. I feel like a strong and powerful woman now, and I've done so much work to get to this place. But still, most of my lived experience was being in a position where I was not respected or listened to. I was encouraged to shut down and be quiet and that's what all women experience.

And the collective – the fact that that's happened to my mother, my grandmother, and it's so clear to me, all the women in my family, apart from me and my sister who have both done a lot of work. This is still the way it's accepted and that's the way it is. It makes me so angry.

Yes, I hear that. It's so powerful recalling our lives as a female. I think that's why you and I both felt so emotional at the beginning of coming together to have this conversation. We know this and we know that what we are doing is changing that, breaking that cycle of the diminishing of who we are.

Absolutely, I truly believe the effects of that. They do go back through the ancestral line as well. It does, it has an effect. I can feel it when I do a particularly powerful piece of work. I've seen it have an impact on my mother even though I haven't spoken to her about it, I know she's felt that. That's what gives me hope.

That's beautiful.

Moving on to this time in your life, did you know what to expect as you began your transition?

I did. Literally, only because of the awareness I've gained over the past few years really. I mean, I haven't spoken about this, but for me part of being a woman was to manage my menstrual cycle. I was on the Pill for a period of time and then I wasn't in a relationship, so I wasn't. But when I met Mark, which was late thirties, even though I'd started, I hadn't started this journey, but I had left finance and was training to be a Hypnotherapist. So I was on that journey of self-discovery. But still, my automatic thought was, 'How can I make this as easy as possible?' So, I started to have the Pill injection so I didn't have to think about any kind of periods, you know. I didn't have any. And initially I thought, 'That's a good thing,' and then I realised that I was just like emotionally feeling completely flat. I felt like completely removed from everything. And that's when I started finding the work of Lisa Lister, Miranda Gray and Alexandra Pope, and I was like, 'Oh my.' That's when I thought, 'What on earth have I been doing?'

I remember saying to Mark, 'I'm stopping,' The word inconvenient was there. I knew it wasn't going to be so easy, but actually it hasn't made any difference really. I thought, 'I can't do this, I'm medicating myself.' I mean what on earth! So, from that point on I started to see the whole of being a woman differently, including Menopause. I think it began from making that decision. And also, I can't remember how many years ago now, probably about four years ago, making the decision to stop dying my hair and it's like, 'What am I doing?' This mask that I've been wearing, and I've always identified with looking young. That was always something I was complimented on, looking like a young girl really. And so, even though physically I wasn't experiencing anything menopausal, I think that was a really major transition for me.

I'm ready, I'm willing to become the older woman that I am. I'm not going to wait, because in my head I'd been telling myself, 'When I get to fifty, I'll stop dying my hair,' and I thought, 'Why am I waiting till fifty?' I don't know what I was thinking! So, I think that was the beginning of it.

But what I'd seen or what I'd experienced of Menopause, again it wasn't really spoken about. The only thing I'd experienced of Menopause, like I said, my grandmother must have been going through Menopause when I was little, when we used to go to her house for lunch on a Sunday. But my mum, she was taking HRT throughout Menopause, so I wasn't aware of any symptoms she was experiencing until she made a decision, for a period of time, to stop taking HRT and the difference was astonishing. It was only a few weeks she stopped taking it for, but she was just like a wild woman. We were all like, 'What on earth?' I remember we were all going out for this big family lunch and everyone was coming. We were meeting at a restaurant on a Sunday and I turned up and my dad was on his own.

I asked, "Where's mum?"

And he said, "She's not coming. She doesn't want to come, she's not coming."

And I rang her and I said, "Mum, what's going on? Don't you want to come and be with everyone?"

And she was just like, "No."

She was very angry during that time and showing it and at the time I was like, 'Oh my goodness, she needs to go back on HRT. What's wrong with her?' That's how I felt at the time and how everyone was reacting to her. But really the stuff that had been building up through her life was exploding out of her. If she was experiencing that now, I would hold space for that in a completely different way, but at the time I was, 'Oh god, there's something wrong with her. She needs to go back on HRT.'

So, that's what I'd experienced of Menopause. That was the only obvious sign of Menopause that I'd seen. And then she did go back on the HRT, and now she regrets that. She had breast cancer a couple of years ago. It was caught very early, but a lot of her friends have had breast cancer as well.

And they were all on HRT?

She says she knows that's what it is. We know our bodies, don't we? I'm so sad mum has had to go through the whole of her life really not feeling that sense of connection. I can see that sadness in her now – so much of her life not being expressed.

I suppose when I was witnessing that and hearing everything that you hear about Menopause, it was, 'Oh my god, that sounds awful.' But because of the journey I've been on over recent years, reconnecting with my body and particularly with my womb, I was kind of looking forward to it to be honest, this transition. I'm at the early stages of it, but I really don't know because it's so mysterious and unique to each woman. I mean obviously there are common things that we experience. It feels like this opportunity to get to know myself more deeply, and that's how I see it.

I hear that. It resonates a lot with me, what you've said. And I think it's really important for other women to know. It's never too late to reclaim all of what you've described, to heal that wounding.

I get what you say about the sadness when you look at your mum. That resonates too because I know my mother didn't fully express herself. And she's dead and gone and she was never able to connect to her womb.

But we can still heal our ancestral wounding and our lineage.

Absolutely. I really don't know with my mum; she goes in and out of being open. There are moments when it feels like she is, and then she shuts down.

And it's her choice, isn't it?

Yes, I know the work I've done around my first bleed, really honouring that experience for myself, allowing my younger self to have that experience and that felt really important for me. So, although I'm talking about the sadness and the anger, I absolutely know that there can be change, even to what we've experienced in the past.

I'm glad you've mentioned your own reclamation of your first bleed. I'd love to come back to that, to hear what you did?

Are there any aspects of your changes so far that you haven't enjoyed, or have been challenging?

I find it's not really challenging; I'm interested now. My cycle was always pretty regular but now I have no idea when I'm going to bleed or how long it's going to last and I can go for a period of two or three months without a bleed, then it'll come. Or having a couple of bleeds within a month. So, I guess that's challenging in a way, because I've really been living in alignment with my cyclical nature, certainly in the last few years and to have known, 'Okay this is how I'm going to feel.' And to know and be aware of that, has been transformational and so beneficial for me. And now, I feel like I'm going to get my bleed, I'm on the edge of it for a couple of weeks. So I'm in that phase for a lot longer – that can be challenging. But also, I'm really curious and interested in that and it's really calling me to connect even more deeply with my body. I can't take it for granted that this is going to happen and this is how I'm going to feel at a certain time. It's like, 'I don't know!'

I really have to listen and trust that and I don't get this all the time. But I do get periods when I get hot, hot flashes and night sweats – not that much, it doesn't happen often, it ebbs and flows. But again, it's felt quite powerful in a way, because I'm in this place of allowing. I'm not, 'Oh my god, this is something I need to manage or medicate or anything.' I'm just like, 'Oh, this is happening,' and I know it's part of a transition and it feels like an initiation, so, bring it on!

So, that's how I'm feeling at the moment. And also because this has been a journey for Mark and me as well since I've been moving into this deeper awareness of my cycle and now moving into Menopause, it's something I've spoken to him about along the way. Just letting him know, the kind of things that might happen and how I might be changing or how I'm expressing myself at times. That helps that he gets that. He doesn't always get it, he's an engineer and is very logical!

But actually, it's interesting, last week, I got my bleed. It was unexpected and it was Day One, it was immediately heavy which is quite unusual, so I was talking to him about it. I woke up the next morning, he asked, "How are you feeling, how's your period?"

And he was like, 'Oh, Day Two is usually the day that you feel most tired.' And I thought, 'Oh, well it is actually.' I thought he does pick this stuff up and he's aware that I'm transforming and changing, that I'm in this transformational journey. So that helps. If I was with someone who didn't get that and wanted to just shut it down all the time and shut me down then I think I would find it incredibly challenging.

It's definitely been a journey for both of us because I remember back when I was saying, "No, I can't have this injection anymore."

And his first response was, 'Oh it's going to be such a pain.' I was on it for about eighteen months.

I thought 'I will have more ups and downs, but that's who I am. So deal with it, basically.' It's been a journey of rediscovery for both of us.

When you look in the mirror now, because you spoke earlier about how your appearance was really central to being a woman all those years ago. So, when you look in the mirror now, if you do, what do you see?

I see me. I feel emotional as I say that, because I don't think I did see me for a long, long time, and that emotion is not surprising, I guess. I do look in the mirror and I love looking in the mirror, into my eyes, because I really do see who I am. I do see an older woman. I was very unaware of that when I first started to allow my grey to come through, I was like, 'Fuck!' I'm older'! I'd been holding it off for all this time. But it feels like my body responded to that – there was relaxation. It was like, okay, I can be who I am, rather than having to hold it all in.

My body is changing. Maybe that's something I'm not completely comfortable with. I think that is actually something that is challenging because I look at my body and it's not that young, slim, youthful body that I never used to have to think about, that was easy for me, and now, yeah, she's changing. I was going to say I don't have the same energy level. I don't feel called, I was always into phases of running and things like that – I just don't feel called to that anymore. Occasionally, I feel like I want to go out and run. Most of the time I don't. I just want to rest more, or maybe do some yoga. Mark and I used to go to the gym together. I really don't feel like doing that at all. So, that's been a big change.

So, I see an older woman. But there is this sense of relaxation and expansion which maybe it doesn't fit with who I was for a large part of my life, but I see this sense of allowing.

Second interview one year later

So, one year on and we're together to complete your interview. I want to begin, after this long gap, by asking what are you experiencing now and do you feel you have shifted into a different space?

Over the summer I was having really intense hot flashes, really intense, one after the other and no bleed since May, about four months without a bleed. Just last week I had a very light bleed and the hot flashes I've noticed are very mild.

I'm not sure, it's an interesting question. I could say, 'Yeah I'm right in it because lots of things are shifting in my life externally.' But I also feel it's the nature of the times we're in (Covid restrictions) and I can see it's still my process, which I can see continuing for another couple of years. It started two years ago when I was first aware of really entering this territory. So, yeah, I really don't think I can say – it's interesting.

I've been thinking a lot about this time and wondering how must it feel to be experiencing your menopausal journey now, in this time when the whole world is experiencing an initiation, a global disintegration. So not only are you dealing with your own disintegration but also that of everything everybody has known.

We have talked about how powerful and how discombobulating that has been, so I wonder if that makes it more difficult to identify for yourself, whether it's The Menopause or whether it's the collective experience?

I'm quite glad, which sounds a bit odd, that this is happening for everyone, that the world is going through this transition at this point while I'm going through my transition. I find it quite comforting really for me. I've known this for a while but what's so clear to me, that just right now, the only thing that we can be sure of, is this continual change. So, I feel that in myself and I'm seeing it externally. I don't think it's making it more challenging. Maybe it is making it more challenging to recognise what's mine, what's collective, but I just feel how we are interconnected with everything, I can really feel that right now. I feel like I am part of this greater whole, this greater transition that's happening. Does that make any sense!?

Yes, it really does. I remember us having a conversation recently and I talked about how I felt I am going through a second disintegration. I'd already experienced menopausal disintegration and come out the other side. And then, this has happened and within this are similar feelings to those I had during the isolation phase of Menopause. That does makes sense to me, because both are an initiation, a death and rebirth experience. We are all letting go of the stuff we thought we knew, what we no longer do. So, yes, what you say makes great sense to me.

It's interesting what you say about it being a comfort to you because everybody is experiencing disintegration. I get that too. Knowing that what I am experiencing, other people are feeling it too and understand.

Yes, I hadn't thought about it like that, but that is exactly how it feels. We're all in this together in our own unique ways. I'm grateful that I'm experiencing Menopause at this time.

What are your feelings about your sexuality and sex as you journey through your Menopause?

This is one area where, I don't want to say I've become disconnected from my sexual self but it feels like it's not so much of a priority, for me, right now. It's taken a back seat, it's a much more inner process for me. I'm talking about it with Mark, we're talking about how we are having less sex at the moment, there's no resentment there. Mark gets that I'm going through this, that I'm experiencing this process – it feels like it's something I've got to do on my own, which is interesting as I've just been talking about being interconnected. But there's this part of it where there's a sexual connection with myself. With Mark, it's there, but it's not at the forefront right now.

It's great that you have a relationship in which you can talk about this openly, I suspect without fear as you said there is no resentment, which makes such a difference doesn't it?

Exactly, yes it does. So much has happened this year – my dad dying, everything that's happening in the world and this sudden shift with us moving back to the UK. Being able to acknowledge that there is so much going on for both of us, that actually, sex is not something that is at the forefront for either of us at the moment. But also, we're still talking about it. It's not like it's something that's been forgotten. It is important, this is really important. So continually checking in around it.

Have you noticed if your relationship is different in other ways? Has the closeness changed?

I feel we have definitely become much closer. Not just this year, we've been on this journey together these past few years. This year we've been much closer. There's a closeness that wasn't there before, this openness, things can pass through much more quickly, and I don't know if that's directly related to us not having sex so often, but I just feel we have become emotionally much closer. I'm not noticing any sense of grief or loss around it. I'm trusting that it will return, I really feel that. So, it's just okay. This is a time when this is how it is. I know that it's still there. I can feel it at times, that sexuality, it's not very often, but it's still there. I have this knowing that it will return, in a different form.

I've experienced a lot around grief and loss this year and continue to. At the moment it doesn't feel like grief for my sexuality or my sexual relationship with Mark. Maybe there is some of that for him though. He hasn't named it as that, but maybe there is, because he's going on a transition as well. It doesn't feel like it's just me. It feels like at the same time, something is shifting for him. So, maybe there is a feeling of loss or grief around losing that part of himself, but that changing from the young man for whom sex was really, really important, and something has shifted around that.

It's so interesting how everything is interconnected. I really feel the reason we are coming back to the UK, it's related to his job, things have changed there. And I feel he is manifesting this changing in circumstances. He's not meant to be in that kind of environment he's been in here (US), not anymore. He's been in that corporate environment, going into the office every day. He's going through this huge transition, all these different layers, it's so interesting!

Yes, it is. When we are in a place of transition, when we are walking in that very wise phase of our life, if we're doing that together as a couple, that's phenomenal, isn't it? It's such a beautiful process to be going through together – differently – but together. Having those channels of communication open. It makes it part of the alchemical process.

Yes. I'm so grateful that I came onto this path and that Mark and I have done the work and that we're able to go on this journey, together.

Absolutely, and it is the time in people's lives when often relationships fall apart because the work hasn't been done, by one, or both. So, it's a blessing when both are allowing those transitions to happen in this magical way.

Exactly, and, not to say there aren't challenges, but I feel if you've got that shared capacity for change and allowing that, it's so, so important.

With the sexual changes, do you feel connected to your womb and yoni and how is the connection different if it is? Not just sexually, but spiritually and in your cyclical life?

I feel I'm continually guided by my womb. It's the part of my body I feel the deepest connection with in terms of how I live my life. The small decisions throughout the day, what I choose to do and how I choose to do it. I feel like she is governing the greater circumstances of my life as well. So, I do feel that connection. At times, it doesn't happen so often, sexually, I do feel that connection and I appreciate it so much more. I notice it more and think, 'Ooh, this is interesting!' What has been interesting, as I'm not having a regular monthly bleed, normally it would be more obvious, the physical connection. I feel like it's more powerful but also more subtle.

Do you feel now, as you don't have that same connection through your monthly blood, do you feel differently in relation to the moon phases?

I definitely notice more now. I always used to, but now it's more intense. The full moon wipes me out. I feel that energy rising, but it can feel a bit like, a bit frenetic and then it can feel like a crash afterwards. Whereas the dark moon and the new moon, I definitely feel more comfortable, much more comfortable in that part of the moon's cycle. That going inwards, slowing down, it feels more spacious. At the full moon I can get stuff done and be connecting with people but it takes a toll on me.

Yup, I hear that. It was absolutely the same for me. It was a real flip on its head. I think when we have that depth of wisdom to connect into the cycle of the moon and understand how it impacts on our energy, we really enable ourselves to respond accordingly in relation to what we do and when we do. It certainly supported me to know when and how I would choose to do specific things in my life. And most importantly when to just 'be,' do nothing. For me that was such a huge part of the alchemy of Menopause, such a precious gift.

So, how do you feel now as you continue your journey ever closer to becoming Crone?

I am genuinely excited about it! I literally sometimes look in the mirror – and this has shifted because I know earlier in my forties I would sometimes look in the mirror and think, 'Oh no,' when I saw my grey hair coming through and how I was looking older, the changes in my body, all those sorts of things. I definitely experienced feelings of loss, loss of my youth. But now, I just feel like, 'Yeah, bring it on!'

I'm going to be fifty at the end of next year, and I'm excited. I used to think I wouldn't know how I'd feel about it, but now I'm, 'YES!' I don't want to wish time away, but I can't wait to move into that stage of my life. I feel pretty ready for it. I look in the mirror now, my face is changing and sometimes I think I look like a different person. It's strange. But I love what I see. And I'm surrounded by such amazing Crone women who are on this amazing journey and are really embracing it. I think that makes a real difference. If my frame for it had been what I'd experienced with the older women when I was growing up, then I would feel very differently. There's such a rising around this at the moment, that I'm excited to be a part of it. I mean it really feels like I am coming into my power.

Ooh yes, I love it.

Another question dropped in as you were speaking. So, you said you are looking forward to coming into your 50s, I have to say I loved my 50s, so let's just take you forward another 10 years, this is not wishing time away, this is just a visioning, looking forward to being 60, when you are going to be post-menopausal. You're in perimenopause now, so you will definitely be 'post' by then! So, just take as long as you need to vision yourself as Crone woman and see what drops in for you.

I see myself on the land, in the land. I feel this is going to be a big part of us coming back to the UK, finding the place where we're meant to be. I can see, I can feel this sense of connection with everything but particularly, I see myself outside with such a strong connection to the land. I have a sense of other women around me; I feel that a part of that is the community that I have and that I'm growing through my work but also it feels there's something around my ancestors as well. It's interesting, because whenever I've done a future self-visualisation, this is who I see, who I've seen and it feels – that word – exciting! It feels really exciting to me that I will get to meet her, be her.

What a time to experience becoming Crone! It is the potency and the power that the world is crying out for.

As you were describing what you were feeling, I was seeing you on the land, a big roaring fire and dancing around the fire with other Crone women, whooping with joy and weaving collective magic and love. That collective voice of Crone saying, "We are here, we are ready, we are radiating love."

Yeah, so much magic in that. And it does feel like a celebration, a real joy in it. So much about right now for me has been about turning what I've been told or what's expected of me, all of this stuff that we've learnt, like literally turning it on its head and that's how I feel about moving into this latter part of my life. This is it, everything else leads to this point.

There's no space for the old stuff!

No, it couldn't be further from the truth. I just feel, I really feel a sense of jubilation. The word that has been coming through recently, which is interesting because the world is so crazy right now, but there is a sense of things are being returned to their natural order, the way things need to be. I'm excited to be part of that.

This message of the book is so, so important to be out in the world.

Thank you Nicola. I have loved having these conversations with you. I feel your story holds such powerful threads of wisdom for other women to become curious about. Such wonderful insights. Thank you.

Reflective Questions

What resonated with you from Nicola's story?

What insights have you gleaned?

What is your biggest takeaway?

LOUISE

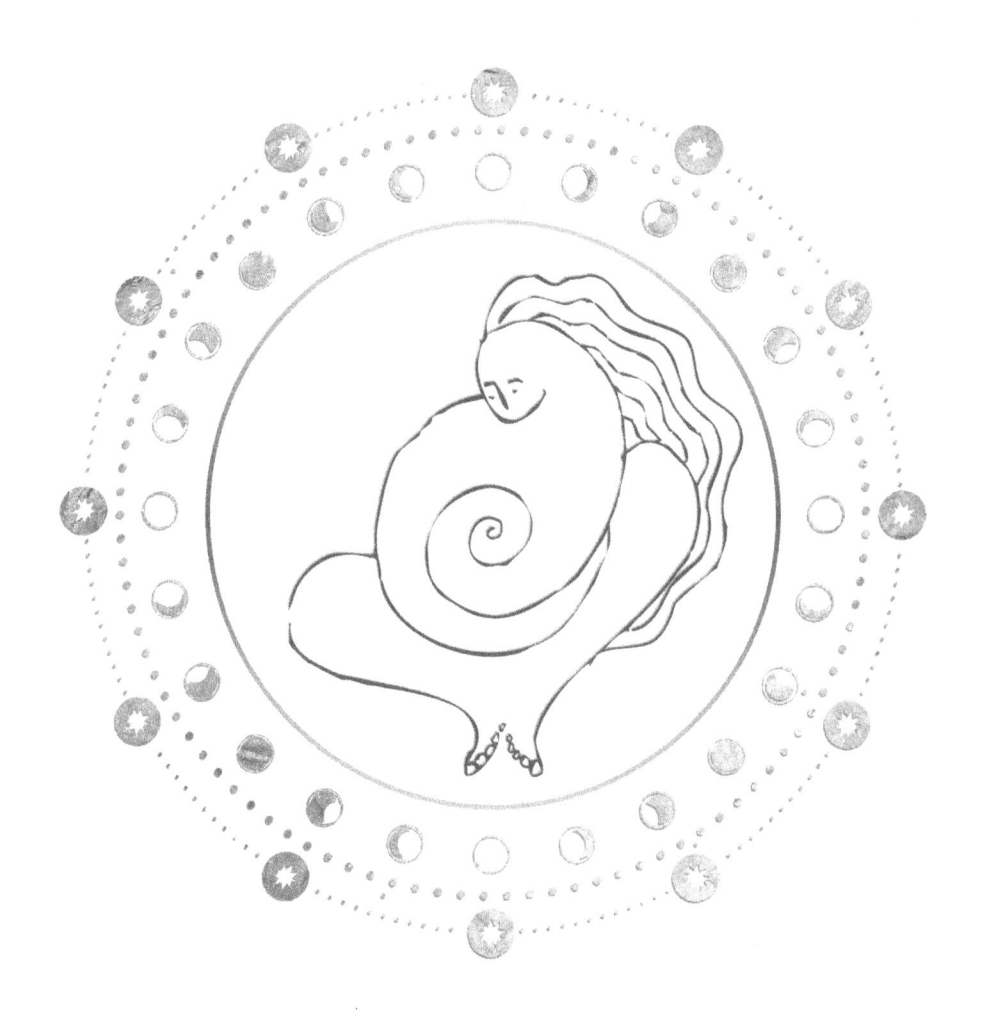

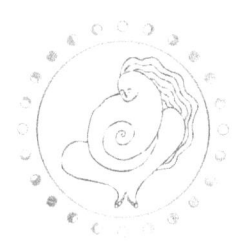

What have you been told or taught about what it is to be a woman? Think back to the first messages you were given by your mother/father/ friends/media.

Things were very positive actually. I liked being female, a woman, a girl. I was the middle child with two brothers either side, so, I was, you know, different. So, in a way, I got more attention. There's suddenly a girl in the middle and I had a good relationship with my dad. My mum said I could charm him, flutter my eyelashes. So already, early on, I was using the feminine wile of that connection between man and woman really.

I enjoyed being girly, I enjoyed it all. What was part of it, very much the 60s generation, I was born in 1959, was that the men were very much in charge, within the family role. The men made the decisions, men were intelligent, you asked them for advice. And the female, the woman, would be doing the cooking and the cleaning and looking after the children. That was generational, but it continues even now.

I think what I was picking up from mum, was that although she was teaching me to look after people, she wasn't very happy with that, she was quite frustrated with that. She wanted a career, I think. And so, there used to be a lot of tension between my mum and dad, with her being stuck with the children, while he worked all day. And then he went off with his amateur acting, so he'd go out in the evenings and Sundays. There was that sense already of how one is balancing all this, being in the female role in a man's world.

I felt my mum's anger and rage about that. I was really so sensitive about that. I felt everything, although I wasn't consciously aware. So, it was – what is the word? – interesting. I loved being a girl but also saw the real downers. For me, there was a sense of needing to be in the masculine energy, especially the mental, the logical. Keeping up with the men, one had to move into more of a masculine energy. There was competing actually, to compete, but again that was very much the 60s and 70s.

There was that horrible phrase, 'You're only a girl.' My brothers would say, 'You're only a girl.' And other people would say it. My husband says it to me now, he says it at his peril, because you know, the rage sets in. He does it as a joke when he wants to wind me up, but I say, "Don't ever say that!"

So, in one sense it was very positive and I loved being girly, being with my girl-friends, doing the make-up, all that, I loved it, the really feminine side. But I had already sussed that I really had to expand my masculine aspect if I was going to be heard.

Yeah, I get what you're saying. Did you ever hear the nursery rhyme that was around when we were children, 'Sugar and spice and all things nice, that's what little girls are made of'?

Yeah, we were there to help. I mean it's that classic thing, at dinner time, I was the one that was laying the table. I mean, where were my brothers? I was the one cleaning and helping mum, where were my brothers? It was always expected that I would do that with my mum, that was definitely the role of the woman. And I remember thinking even then, 'This isn't fair. I don't understand this.'

But I was always – I've done the work since – a 'People Pleaser.' I wanted to please people so they would give me attention and love. But actually underneath, it was what the role had to be and it was quite clear. Although interestingly enough, my granny, on my mum's side, she was a Cartologist, and if she'd been born in a different generation, I feel she wouldn't have had children. She wasn't really a maternal type, my mum and my aunt talked about this. She did have children, but she wasn't maternal. Her career came first, she was a highly intelligent woman. Then my mum, from that family set up, she then walked into the role of, 'I'll give up my job as soon as I'm married, and then I start having children and looking after them.' I think I had both didn't I? – the two role models – but the balance is out of kilter.

Yes, it's interesting that you use the word balance. I was going to ask you that question, specifically about your masculine and feminine energy. Do you feel you had a balance of the feminine and masculine at some point, and did it become unbalanced as you grew from child to woman because of the role models you grew up in?

Mmmm, that's interesting, I think I've struggled all my life with that balance actually. I think when I'm in a situation where I think I've got to be the strong one, I've got to be the one that provides, I've got to be the one sorting and organising, then I very quickly get into that left hand side of the brain, that masculine energy and I then stop listening to myself, to my true self, to my feminine intuitive, creative side. You know, I'm not writing, I'm not being creative, I'm doing all those things one has to do. And I think I can get very into that because it's been a very strong part of when I was young, needing to keep up. My brother went to Oxford, my father was incredibly intelligent, and so was my mum, but she felt left out of the conversation and I could see this going on. I kind of wanted to be almost more like dad than mum actually. But then having said that, I could have been an academic student, studied and been in my masculine head. But I wasn't. So, I really think, that when I was younger the balance was quite good. I think when I got to my late twenties and thirties that's when I got into my psychic, intuitive work. So, then I was beginning to get that kind of balance.

How do you think those various messages impacted on you at that point in your early twenties, when you started to become aware of your psychic gift?

That was actually when I was a small child, at puberty when it often starts, but I'd already closed it down, which was fear-based. My mum was quite psychic but she wasn't going there, she didn't like it, it was not pleasant for her. So, she switched it off. Later-on in life she said to me, "I'm not going there in this life; I'm not doing it."

But she was very interested in what I was doing. She was worried for me, she went back into her fear. And then she saw that I was actually perfectly fine, this is who I am, and she then went, 'Ooh, okay' and I would tell her about what I was doing.

You mentioned puberty and how that was your awakening to your psychic abilities. What do you recall about your first bleed?

It's funny isn't it? It started to be, that now you're having periods, it was something you just had to bear, just had to get on with it. It was like an inconvenience, so it was never embracing or celebrating being a woman. In so many cultures, it was, 'Yes, you're bleeding, so here are some towels and get on with it. If you don't feel well, just tell me. Here's a hot water bottle.' And that was really it.

I was a very late starter, about fourteen, one of the last in my school. Some were about eleven. My best friends had boobs at twelve and kept asking, 'Haven't you started yet?' and I'd say, 'No.' But no-one still really talked about it. That's what's interesting, we didn't really talk about what happens. I just knew it was probably something really awful because they would feel very unwell and take the day off school and I didn't like being unwell. So, it was actually something not to embrace for me and mum didn't talk about it.

When I started, I found the blood in the toilet and I thought I was dying. I thought, 'Oh my God, I'm bleeding, I'm losing blood.' And then I thought, 'Oh, could it be?' So, I went straight to mum and she said, "Oh, yes, that's your period. Okay, have some towels. Take some Paracetamol if you don't feel well."

I think I had the day off school, so bless her she was looking after me. But there wasn't any kind of acknowledgment of the transition. In the West, we don't do this, unless you're very lucky with your mum. I mean she didn't go, 'Oh my goodness, we don't talk about it,' We were open, but we *didn't* talk about it!

How did she refer to your menstruation? My mum called it the, 'The Curse.'

Oh yes, yes, 'The Curse,' I'd forgotten that. I mean what is that about! It means it's a dread, a fear and inconvenience.

I remember having to go through my calendar to work things out, like if I was going to have a tennis match, seeing I'll probably have my period, it was all negative.

That's interesting what you've just said about the calendar and that you were tracking it, but still from the perspective of it being an annoyance. Whereas, lots of young women I know, now use a menstrual cycle calendar or an App on their phone. Not because they regard it as an inconvenience but because they celebrate it and they positively plan their weeks according to where they're going to be in their cycle. It's so different.

Oh yeah, so different, how wonderful. It's embracing that part of us; it just is part of us and it's hugely important. And it's that classic thing isn't it, that nobody talked about it? Certainly, I didn't talk about it to my dad.

Even when I was at school, I went to Eastbourne Co-educational College and you never ever talked about it at all. And it was all that, 'Oh she's got her period.' It was an embarrassment. Looking back on it, it's really sad. Again, it's about being in a man's world. If they had them every month, my goodness wouldn't we be talking about it! You'd be hearing all about it – how difficult it is for them etc.

Did you feel a need to hide your sanitary products and when you were bleeding, from your dad and brothers?

Yes, we didn't keep any towels in the toilet at home. They were in a drawer in my bedroom. Never kept them lying around. And even at school, we kind of talked about it and I was using sanitary towels, because that's what mum used. She did use Lillets too, but she was of the generation that thought you shouldn't use tampons if you were a virgin. I didn't know she thought that, I just thought I shouldn't use them because they're bad for you, they're just bad for you, which of course they are! Her wisdom was telling her one thing, but it was coming from a different consciousness.

When I went to Eastbourne College, these girls were very independent people, you know. I'd never left home. And I had an accident one day, I do remember this, I was just walking back from classes to the house where we all lived, and one of the older girls came up behind me and said,

"Don't worry. I'm just going to stand behind you, just keep going, just keep going. You've just had a little accident."

My blood had gone through the sanitary towel, and I just remember being absolutely mortified. I wasn't going to leave the house now, I was leaving the whole school, you know! And so, my friends took me in hand and said, "Why are you still wearing sanitary towels, this is ridiculous, you're a young, modern woman?"

And it knocked me and I said, "Oh, no, no I can't."

I think I had tried once myself and I found it difficult.

They put me in the toilet cubicle and told me not to come out until I had it up there! It was quite traumatic actually.

In a way, it was kind of liberating for me, because I hated using sanitary towels.

I was always worried about the smell. I didn't have a sister to talk to, and my mum never really talked about it and I couldn't talk to her about tampons anyway. I had no-one at home really to talk to. So, in a way my school friends were like my sisters, taking me in hand and going, "For goodness sake, don't suffer like this. Just get the tampon in."

And it took about twenty minutes and they all sat outside the toilet and told me how to do it. They weren't in my face, but they sat there until I had managed to. And I was so, so joyful that I had actually managed to do something that at that time we all thought was really helpful. And so, I actually felt very supported in that moment. Thinking back on it now, there were about two or three of them there helping me, so it was like a women's circle, like a women's support group, who were there outside the toilet waiting for Louise to get to grips with a tampon. I do think of that with some fondness, although it was traumatic to begin with. At first, I thought, 'How dare you, how dare you do this!' But I knew they were there, and I wanted to help myself.

How did you usually feel about your menstrual blood?

I'm not good with blood. It was a difficult thing. I used to feel very faint, so losing the blood, seeing it in the toilet pan and on the towels used to make me feel *ugh*. Again, that's to do with fear and other things that I wouldn't even have connected with at that time. It didn't help at all that I was often not in my body. I'd rather be up here (indicating to above her head) where it's light, and being in my body feels heavy and quite difficult and so I have to work quite hard to be in my body. So of course, with the blood, it was another way of me going, 'Whoa, I need to come out of here.'. But if it had been embraced, if it had been a positive aspect, I could have come back into my body. And funnily enough, when I was doing the womb meditation on my own just now, I felt, 'Wow, this is so grounding,' like coming back into my body, back to my womb and be truly back in.

That's wonderful to hear the meditation, connecting to your womb, has helped you to feel grounded and in your body.

Have you considered how your experience of menstruating impacted on you as you approached your Menopause years?

Yeah, just try and ignore it, not being fully in the body! It was like, just get on with it. It was the real stoic, middle class family thing, you just get on with it.

You don't complain and you just suffer it. In silence actually. Until I looked back on that I didn't know that was what I was doing. But I had been told, 'You just got on with it.' I mean you could talk about it and complain about it, but there was a great sense, with my mum, to be very practical, very straight forward. You just get on with it.

So, I think the Menopause too was, you just get on with it! It happens, and you deal with it, that would be the word, you *deal* with it. So, I don't think I was prepared and I certainly didn't prepare, and mine was quite early because, I don't know if this had anything to do with it, I lost my ovary from having an ovarian cyst. I had it after Mountview (Drama School) and they operated on me. And at no time did they say they were going to take my ovary out if they had to, at no time, and I was only around twenty-two years old.

So, I wake up, and this doctor – I do remember it now, my mum was furious about this – I woke up, I was groggy from the drugs, and the doctor came and sat on my bed and said, "The operation went very well," and he started to tell me, "Although it was a water cyst, it was benign, but it was too large, so we had to take the whole ovary out."

And I remember thinking, 'Sorry? What? What did you say?'

The doctor said, "We have removed the whole ovary. But you still have one, you have one, you can get pregnant if you want." And he walked off.

I remember my mum coming the next evening and I was thinking, it was kind of like, I took it on a conscious level and thought, 'Oh right, okay.' Then I could feel, even then, that absolute shock of, 'What have they done?'

I've talked to other women who have only one ovary. You don't have a period every month. The other ovary goes, 'It's your turn now. Oh, nothing's happening. Okay I'll do it again.'

And I had a sense, other people have said that they have had the same experience, that it's almost as if they're (the remaining ovary) going to run out of eggs, or they've worked double time. So, bless it. I have blessed my ovary that's still here and the ovary that went.

I became menopausal when I was about forty-seven years old. I started quite early. It was quite surprising, but then it seemed to be quite logical really. And actually, I was very lucky, I didn't have very heavy periods, they were quite light all my life, and I feel thankful for that because of the whole blood thing. I've had my moments, nothing too dramatic. They just kind of petered out.

But then, talking about it, just horrendous stuff went on.

No preparation, no viewing it at all. This just happens and it came early, so none of my friends who were my age, nobody comparable with me, no-one had started at all. So, I was the first of my group – and, why do women not talk about Menopause?

We were all trained not too weren't we. There was Menopause Month on Radio 4, recently, I don't know if you were aware of that?

I was, 'Yeah, that was brilliant.'

I used to listen to Women's Hour regularly and The Menopause has been a theme from time to time but largely with a focus on HRT or about the symptoms and still largely carrying a negative perspective of it.

Yes, I agree.

Nobody has spoken about the alchemy of it, this incredible transformation that's bringing us to being Crone, to that place in our life and in the world where we are so powerful and so healing. The world needs Crones!

Absolutely, we are the wise women, who stand in many cultures, who are then celebrated. We have such a lot to offer. And as you say, I've heard programmes that talk about HRT and nobody talks about how horrendous HRT can be and what on earth you're putting in your body. And also, again the negative, talking about the hot flushes and so women are already into fear before they even reach Menopause. It's something again either to, 'Oh my goodness, let's medicate this as fast as I can,' or to push it away and just get on with it, rather than, 'Right, here we go!'

Do you have any recollection of your mum's experience of Menopause?

I asked her when I was going through such a bad time, I asked, "Mum, what happened to you?"

And she said, "Well, it's funny you know, I don't really remember."

And we worked it out that my dad died at 52 and mum was 50. And she said, "I think I was just beginning my Menopause when your father died and I just have no idea, I don't remember really. I think I had some hot flashes; I don't really remember it being too bad."

But then she was dealing with the grief at such an early age. She wasn't fully present with it at all.

That's really interesting, because part of our transition, part of that alchemy is grief. The grief of losing what we were, what we understood, a shedding. So that must have been quite something for your mum to be holding the grief for the loss of her life partner and the grief of her own disintegration.

It may be that it was all happening together and she just wasn't aware of it. Whether it increased the grief, I don't know, I guess she was just in it. Again, she said, "I just had to get on with it. I had three children."

My younger brother was only 14, so I think she just put her head down. So, there was no family hand down of what happened. No, nothing at all.

And that's another piece that I think is interesting for our generation to explore. What you're describing is very typical. My experience is of the healing that happens when we reclaim our lost or forgotten transitions. The healing happens not just for us but for our lineage, our ancestral story.

Do you feel that it depends on your belief system? We are all one, so as we heal our self, we're healing others? In my work there is such a huge sense around ancestral healing. We can leave past life to one side. That's another level, but at the moment ancestral healing feels so huge. It's genetic, and as we heal ourselves, we are healing the line, past, present and future.

Mmm, I got goose bumps as you said that. To be honest that's what the alchemy of my Menopause has been, the connection not only to my ancestors but to the Earth as well. Your voice, what you're expressing now, all the voices of the women who are contributing to this book, I believe it's so important they go out into the world as part of the healing process.

The intention, setting my intention, is about that healing, releasing and speaking my Truth for myself and for others.

You've mentioned Menopause symptoms a few times. How have you felt about those symptoms you have had?

Okay, I did really, really suffer. I started with these hot flashes that just would come up the body and I was just like an oven, just like I was about to explode, absolutely explode. I've had really bad one's for about six years, and they would make me feel so unwell that I would get to the point of not knowing who I was. I obviously had moved out of my body, so I would feel dizzy, feel sick. And the sweat, I would be dripping from head to foot and I'd have to be doing this (wiping sweat from upper lip), everywhere, just everywhere, legs, arms, everywhere.

It was in the night as well, I had night sweats. So, I was on towels and they would happen, at the peak, about every two hours – day and night – and how long can you keep going that way? Just exhausted. I said to my husband, "I haven't had children but I assume this is what sleep deprivation is like."

Trying to deal with something physical but you're not able to rest. You're trying to get through it. I couldn't concentrate, I couldn't remember. At the height of it I'd taken on a full-time job in an investment company. I look back on it and I wonder why I did that. But I know it was to give me confidence to then step out into the world – somebody believed in me and valued me.

I was still doing my holistic work and training. But it was very important those two years in the investment company, to be really valued. I really appreciate that. But of course, it was incredibly full on. I was Director. It was at the time of recession. It was really tricky, huge financial negotiations, all sorts of things were going on. I was really enjoying aspects of it, but I had to be on it, top notch. I'd be in a meeting that I'd called, and they'd all look at me and go, 'Right, yes Louise, so?' And I don't know what day it is. 'Why are we here?' And I'd just see people staring at me and I had no idea what I was meant to be doing. It just got worse and worse.

I felt very unwell, I felt depressed, I had a really bad time. I had problems with my sciatic nerve. I was going to a Chiropractor. I went to my Homeopath, an amazing intuitive Homeopath. She gave me remedies, but it really was getting worse and worse. I just felt like I was losing my mind. I completely lost myself, I didn't know who I was. I would have these surges of rage. I can keep very supressed, 'Louise doesn't get angry, she doesn't lose her temper.' Of course I *do*, but I may not do it publicly. But I'd have a real surge, whoomph! – and I'd go, 'Oh my goodness!'

Of course, looking back, I think, 'What power was that!' And thank you for that because in your book (*Take Off Your Armour*), you wrote about hot flushes, 'That is your power,' and I really wish I'd read that when I was going through it because actually, I could have shifted it so strongly and as such a positive aspect. It was my lion roaring and I *love* that, I love that – thank you.

But I didn't have that perspective then. I had real ups and downs and feeling like I can't cope. I can't cope with the world. So, I understand why people get suicidal with it.

For me, therein lies the sadness really. All of that happens for so many of us in the way you're describing because we have not been told, or taught, or shown, that all of that is our power, it's our healing.

I'm really interested to ask you, as a psychic, someone who's very connected to intuition – actually as I'm saying that, I think I get what it may have been for you, the disparity? Because The Menopause on one level is very physical, on another level, it's so other worldly, a place of visioning and dreaming, out of the body – did you feel any of that?

I think because I was so exhausted physically and was just trying to keep going, the classic family – keep going – that I was less in connection. It almost shifted me out, because in a way I wanted to deny it, because I didn't want to be suffering. And also, because sleep deprivation for me was a nightmare. Then I start to be in another world anyway. So, unfortunately, it was kind of pushing me out of my body, rather than connecting. But, if I think about it, it was at that time that I started to train in my Spiritual Counselling, although I'd already trained as a Channeler and was working a little bit.

I've shifted and developed unbelievably fast in these last ten years. I have, I've just acknowledged that right now. Looking back, I have stepped into my power. I am doing the things I want to do – I am, yaaaay – so hell, that's amazing! I hadn't actually acknowledged that at all before now.

I can feel the power of your energy as you say that Louise.

But it had been such a struggle. How could I possibly have done anything?

And in those couple of years, holding those two years of hell, the Universe did lead me and actually I left the corporate job. It wasn't serving me anymore. It had served me to begin with but I wanted to leave. And the Menopause pushed me out of it actually, which was absolutely right. So, intuitively, it served its purpose and I'm leaving, I'm out. Usually, I stay far longer than I should, and I just went, 'No, I'm not doing this again, I'm out.'

I reasoned at the time that I couldn't cope, I couldn't deal with the job. I wasn't adding value, I wasn't earning my money as it were. But actually, of course, no, it was, 'Thank you very much, but now I'm moving onto the spiritual healing work that I want to do.' So, I gave up that job and from that point I went, 'Right, I'm now a counsellor.' So, it accelerated my psychic work, that's the word, that's it.

I'm going to take some time after this conversation to really, fully integrate these realisations. I do totally trust that part of who I am, that everything is exactly as it's meant to be and however much I rale and try to control, whatever I might be trying to do, I have to trust that. When I look back on my life, everything, every little thing, every little piece of the extra piece, the bricks in the wall, the foundations that makes me exactly who I am today and what I'm doing; and it's all perfect.

Yes, I agree, everything that goes before brings us to where we are.

It doesn't feel that on the way, does it? I asked so much, 'What am I doing?' The number of times in my life I've gone, 'What on earth am I doing here? How have I got here?' But it's all part of the purpose, it's part of my Soul. When I'm listening, I'm incredibly wise – I know where I'm going – but not consciously all the time!

How did you manage those challenges you've described?

So, there was the mental fog, the physical symptoms and then I decided to try HRT, which I really didn't want to do. But I thought, 'I can't continue like this,' and I tried some of the herbal remedies but it just wasn't happening. It was just really interesting, making decisions, watching my choices. I was being pushed to what was important. Although I got halfway there by leaving the job, I was not looking after myself physically. I don't think so. So, I did take HRT for three months and it became obvious I was completely allergic to it because after three months, my whole face blew up. I had problems breathing at one point and then I was getting horrendous viruses and colds. I see a homeopathic doctor – I have always used homeopathy and she said, "Louise, you are having an allergic reaction. Get off it now."

And I went, 'You are so right.' My immune system had crashed, completely crashed with HRT in my system. So, I only had it for three months.

Interesting enough, in those three months, my mental abilities came back and the mental fog didn't reappear. I reckon it took two years to get the HRT out of my system and for me to fix my immune system. I am a very sensitive person anyway with drugs so, it probably wasn't the best thing for me! I do remember my doctor saying when I went back to tell her I was coming off of it, that I wasn't okay. And she said, "Well Louise, I would not suggest that you do that, I have got nothing else to offer you. You are either going to suffer or just take the HRT. So, I think the HRT is the better option."

And she knew that you were having the allergic reaction?

Yeah. But I couldn't *prove* that. So, I thought, 'Oh, where's that support, you know, woman to woman?' She was my age; she was going through it too. In fact, we get along very well and we are kind of in a mutual appreciation society. Normally she listened. But this one was really bad. She thought it was alright, okay for me to be having all these problems and still take it. Where's her thinking in that?

Well, that's so interesting, isn't it? Because the fact that she was a woman of the same age and experiencing Menopause for herself. I would guess from her response to you saying, 'Look, the HRT is not working,' and her believing you should stay on it, that she perhaps, was not experiencing the alchemy of Menopause. Her view and experience were medical, a medicalised approach to The Menopause. So, having a conversation with you to explore other options, to be open to something non-medical was maybe outside her experience? And that reiterates for me how as women, we have been sucked into this vortex of thinking The Menopause, like pregnancy, like childbirth, like menstruation needs to be medicalised and controlled.

And take a pill and shut up basically, which was the male dominant view, especially in the 1950s and 1960s. Take a pill for your anxiety. I've been suffering from anxiety attacks. I've had them in the past. I've been having them over the last two years. And it still feels like the 1950s and 1960s with being told, 'Here's a little pill for you, you'll feel so much better,' and still with the side effects.

I think it's that patriarchal, archaic attitude of, 'Be quiet, you neurotic woman!' It happened to my mum.

The rational masculine side of my brain was going, 'You know this is practical, this is logical, this is what they give you. Take it.' It was really very strange because she is such a good counsellor doctor as well. She is very good and she really likes me. We have a sort of appreciation of each other's talents and skills.

I did stop taking HRT. I didn't see her for about a year after that. For me, my reaction to that was really, 'I am alone here.' I just had to come back to self again, which is where we all come back to, I think.

So, it has been a long journey for me. Some people just don't suffer from Menopause, do they? They don't, they say, 'Oh, yes, I don't really remember how the Menopause was for me.' Or somebody said to me, "Well, I was determined my Menopause would not affect me and it didn't."

But I really suffered and I thought, 'It's part of me.' Some people have had a lot of children and often then Menopause can be hugely emotional, you know, from being mother earth, the mother, to suddenly losing that aspect of themselves. So, there is that grief and that loss. That was an interesting one for me, because I thought, 'Oh well, then perhaps this won't affect me *because* I don't have children.' And, then I thought, because I haven't had children, that's a huge thing for me, because suddenly it's gone and so perhaps there's that grieving or that loss of *not* having children.

Yes, I get that. I think whether you've had children or not, we all have or have had a womb and she is our centre of creativity. For many women, by the time they reach Menopause, they have perhaps had a hysterectomy. But we still have our energetic centre of creativity, whether that was being creative through being a mother or through our work or through our home. So, whatever our experience has or hasn't been, it comes at last to the Menopause. It is that point in our lives where we are asked to look at all of that, whatever it has been. To look at all of that and what unfolds and what that means as we disintegrate from who we thought we are.

Yeah. And there is that loss.

Absolutely, grief and loss is massive for so many women I have talked with.

Being able to create through our wombs, as you say, creating, I *have* been creative in other ways. That's interesting. I am not good with loss. I find it very difficult to process. I hang on to it and I suffer quite a lot. So, I just wondered whether that was all going on during Menopause.

It's interesting, as we have these conversations. I hear you say loss is difficult for you and you expressed earlier about the loss of your ovary, and how it brought up the loss around not having children. And then when Menopause arrived for you, you were asked to look at that loss again.

Of course, yeah. We need to do it.

I'm interested that you have used the word 'suffered', that you feel you suffered with the Menopause. Do you want to speak about that?

Yeah. What did I mean by that, 'suffered'? That *is* interesting. Maybe there is some guilt somewhere about not having children. That's just coming in now as we speak. What is it? I'm just feeling into that.

I feel that in the past, in past lives, I've had lots and lots of children. I felt very strongly that this life was to really be for *my* time and also to be a 'mother' in so many other ways, be creative in all those other different ways.

Something's really coming through on this.

I want to explore that, what do I mean by that, suffering? Is it just giving myself excuses – I can do what the hell I want? Or not follow the line that everyone expects, expectation from families, and mothers and parents and other people sometimes, in my experience. So, it's an interesting one. I felt so clearly, whenever I visited each past life, it was not children I wanted in this lifetime and I knew that it was not going to happen. Perhaps on some Soul level, with that mother within me, there was a bit of guilt about not having them. Especially as I got older. I thought, 'Wouldn't it be so lovely now to reap the rewards of having children and seeing how they are supportive to parents?' But then, not every child is. So, it's all that stuff still going on, that processing of decisions to have children or not. So, it's all very interesting, the suffering. Yeah. I need to look at that more about what that means.

Ooh, yes, that sounds like a potent piece to explore further.

There is that sense of this constant progression of which I'm doing as I have continued to do my spiritual work and a much deeper letting go, really getting through the grief they (past life children) have gone.

I still get hot flushes. I can sit here and suddenly go like, 'Phew, hot. I need to take my jumper off!' I can get them at night too, but it's nothing compared to how it was during that time I talked about before. That's 12 years ago. So, I would say, I had them really badly for quite a number of years.

I'm having one now.

Oh, there we go. Yeah. Just talking about it!

Tuning in. You're connecting into the energy, I often get it when I am working with somebody, one to one, or if I'm starting a workshop, in the first hour. That's because energetically I'm shifting things through, I am moving into more spaciousness and energy. I'm working on a higher vibration. So, it *is* something that helps connect us, raising our vibration.

Well, I think so. Yeah. I think sometimes it's shifting out and sometimes it's bringing it in. I think it's interesting to kind of note how that feels as it's happening.

I think for me it was letting go. It was clearing out to begin with. Yes, it was to begin with and I think, I resisted it on some level. I think it was a resistance to it also as an age thing with me. I am incredibly vain! I have always looked younger than I have been. Not so much now, I mean in the last 10 years, for goodness sake!

I don't do age, and therefore I don't expect other people to stop treating me differently because of how I look.

I absolutely agree with you, the last 10 years, from 50 approaching 60, I've really aged. I'm like you, I always looked much younger than I was, so it's been a surprise to see the aging over that period of time. It felt sudden, quick.

This leads us on to the next question, when you look in the mirror, what do you see?

I see a wise Soul actually, and I see a child. I have always connected to child. Something that was coming through in the last 10 years, when I connect with somebody, I connect with their child first and if I can sense that child,

I know I'm going to really connect with them. Not on a professional basis but on a friend-to-friend basis or people that I meet, I sense whether there is going to be a connection, whether we can be friends, if there is that sense of the child in them. I was completely unaware of that when I look back. Now, it's a heart-to-heart connection – can I come and play with you? Can you come and play with me? And that fun sort of connection.

So, there is still child in me. It's strong and that's why I grieve over loss. The child finds it really hard. So, I see the child, when I look in the mirror.

What else do I see? I see someone with quite a lot of pain sometimes and hurt. I can't quite work out the world sometimes; there's a bit of confusion. I can't work this out or I am lost, or there is a sense of working and figuring things out.

I see both masculine and feminine. I have got a quite strong masculine side; I see them both. I do see a balance in that, but I see a female face. I see Louise.

But what's interesting is that I have never been good with identity. Being an actress, that was so difficult, and I think that's why I was not perhaps as successful as I might have been. I never quite knew who I was or how other people saw me.

I see a woman of equal, a woman. She is 61. There are some laughter lines here and there, some pain and disappointment here. I go straight into the eyes and the Soul. I love to think about that.

I love that you have answered in that way. When I first asked myself that question, I answered it on a very physical level.

That actually really confirms for me how I have difficulty grounding and being in the physical realm. I'm seeing myself in a spiritual aspect, my physical is floating.

Let's explore that a little bit then, because I remember that you said that you've left your body a lot throughout your life. So, how do you see yourself as a 61-year-old woman in the physical sense, in a grounded, 3D sense?

Just older. I see my eyes disappearing. They are sort of who I am; there's less definition. But all that doesn't worry me anymore because I think, as we really connect to that spiritual aspect and Soul, this physical, it's not important. I didn't get that in my 20s and 30s. I saw my boobs as too small and my waist as too big. And I got to be an item. I was always having to lose that 'extra stone' at drama school and goodness knows what I was trying to be, under nine stone because there was that pressure. Losing the weight in the summer, then putting it on in the winter. So, I was physically kind of aware of that then and with the Menopause, I put on a stone and a half over the space of four years.

And then I had a heart diagnosis, where they said I had the beginnings of heart disease and that my cholesterol was up. I thought, 'Right, I have to really take hold of this,' because my father died of heart disease.

So, then I lost two stone within two years and I have never put it back on. I'm eating, I mean, for goodness sake, eating during lockdown, let's face it! I shouldn't be checking, but you know, I have been eating far more and I'm not putting the weight back on. I feel when I was a teenager, weight-wise, I felt light. It felt good. It wasn't ungrounded for me funnily enough. I felt more ungrounded being heavy, which is a very weird thing. Now I feel as I naturally should be.

Do you think perhaps it might be because, you said early on, it doesn't matter to you anymore? Because it doesn't worry you now, you don't have that concern about what you look like physically, so actually you can now feel comfortable?

Yeah, and I think I have let it go. I think I've let go of the worry of keeping, holding on and holding off. Also, I think letting go, perhaps there's been real fearful stuff going on the last two years. But somehow, putting on weight is to ground us, is to protect us around the solar plexus. So, energetically it's shielding us, putting that protective layer from the world and possibly that's what I was doing through that transition. I was so unsure of myself and losing myself in the whole menopausal stuff and what it meant and the physical symptoms. I don't think I was eating anything *more*, but all this weight just kept coming on.

Yes, I'm bringing me into the body. So, all of my physical symptoms that I have in this life, I'm just going to have to be in this physical body. I'm fine. I'm here. I've let go of all that stuff. I am spiritual, I am who I am. More myself now I have allowed it. I've let go of what people expect of me or think of me or who *they* think I am.

It doesn't matter anymore.

And that is the gift The Menopause brings to us.

Yeah. I think for me, I felt very weak and kind of not here and existing within the Menopause, losing parts of oneself, and how other people then see you as you are getting older. As you say, that transition is so important to really *earth* yourself into 'Hey, this is me. It is the gift!'

I choose which friends I talk to about my spirituality, which is fine. I may not talk about it anymore with some friends, but it's fine. I choose them, it's fine. Everyone is on their own journey and I am on mine as long as people respect that. I have got far less, what is the word? Tolerant, far less tolerant of disrespectful people.

Yes! I see that as another gift of The Menopause. We seem to have this ability to say strongly and clearly, 'I'm not accepting that.' Setting boundaries is far easier now.

Yeah, I think it does give clarity. I think it forces you to find yourself, because losing who you are and basically all these changes, with lack of sleep and lack of mental clarity, you have to find a way through. I remember saying to my husband, that I didn't know who I was anymore. I really had lost me.

There was fun too. So, it does give you that gift. You have to work your way through that, which is definitely a gift. It's that sense of freedom, of letting go of all the stuff we have had from huge society pressure for women. Whether it was to look size zero or trying to look young, or whether to have children or get married or to look really powerful and strong in business; all these dreadful roles and stereotypes that we spend so much time trying to duck and dive them.

Doesn't matter anymore.

That's the potency and the power, isn't it?

So, let's look at sex and sexuality as a post-menopausal woman. How do you feel about that? What's changed? What's been let go of? What's come in?

I think the sadness is, that through all those changes, our sexual relationship, my husband really suffered on that one because I just didn't feel like it. The idea of making love with hot flushes going on all the time, it became horrible and I didn't want him to touch me anymore. It affected our relationship – that's been hard. The physical changes, I mean, having a cervical smear now is horrendous. It wasn't actually quite so bad last year. I had one last year and it was not actually quite as bad, which is encouraging.

Our relationship has changed as well. I mean, we were never like rabbits! We were quite matched, you know, in our sexuality. So, making love was something which was about being together, about making love. Our relationship wasn't always about the actual intercourse. We are best mates. So yes, it has been rocky, but on the other hand it is part of that relationship I think, as well. Because relationships do change. It becomes a different thing. Sex becomes not so essential. It's probably not the same for the male. What's essential is being together and being close – that can be intimate. But yes, it has changed.

Is that something that you have been able to talk about together? Or did it feel terribly taboo and difficult to talk about how you felt differently about that physical connection?

I am somebody who always thinks, if I just ignore it, it will go away. So, to be honest, yeah. We didn't really talk about it. I just thought, 'Oh, this will get better,' and then I think I got quite impatient with myself because it wasn't that I stopped feeling I wanted to make love. It was just that it was all just physically, 'Oh God,' you know, it was just too much. The hot flushes really diminished our sex life. Feeling so hot and towels over you, it just wasn't sexy.

I think also for me it was putting on that weight that I had. I did suddenly have boobs, I had a cleavage, oh my God, you know, that was amazing! And in a way I could enjoy that a bit. But I know I felt so fat, so big and sweaty and hot and I am quite a smelly person when I get hot. I began to feel the change of how sexy I felt and what makes me feel sexy. And I didn't feel sexy.

Now as a post-menopausal woman, as a woman in her Crone phase of life, how do you feel about sex and sexuality?

It's not top of my list. Does that make sense? It's lovely, but we don't very often, but when we do it's great. I think to be honest, my husband would much rather it was much more often but he is incredibly respectful about it. I mean, he's amazing really. And also, for him, he's slowed down too. He doesn't have the same kind of stamina, so it's a different thing. So, we just have to kind of go along that journey together on that.

We do talk about it now but probably not enough. We probably don't talk about it too much because it's sometimes a bit upsetting. It's been upsetting because I don't want to say, 'Look, I don't need it so much.' Because it sounds like I don't fancy him. And then my husband gets into a real thing about me not fancying him, but I *do* fancy him, and being intimate is great. But the act of actual intercourse, it's not comfortable either sometimes. I don't know, I just don't need it as much, but I want to sometimes. There's no reason why we can't just continue as we have always done. I have to say, talking to people, it seems that a lot of people just don't have sex. Young people too.

I think my husband would say, he would like it more often, yes. Far more. It's not that I don't feel sometimes really sexy. It's very hard to explain, isn't it?

It's a really interesting piece about sex and sexuality and I think it's something that isn't spoken about enough between friends, let alone between couples, but between friends, between women. I think it's a subject that for many of us still feels very uncomfortable. When I asked that question of myself, I thought, right, I am going to put this question to each of you, this is really important. I did think, 'Okay, how is this going to feel for other women to answer?' And I honour all of you so deeply for allowing me to ask you. I wonder if that's also generational, because although we were born in the sixties, we weren't in the sixties as young women but we were part of that sexual revolution and I think it all became something quite different as we became young women.

A number of women have said that it's uncomfortable for them to have actual intercourse. But that they do still sometimes feel like they would like an orgasm. So, do you ever self-pleasure?

Yes, I do. Again not very often, but yes, I will do that. And then that is an interesting one, because I hadn't realised, when you do have the orgasm, it's like that kind of build-up, like the hot flushes, which I kind of hadn't connected before. In a very *different* way, but it's pleasurable the hot flush in orgasm, bringing the energy through. So, that's a good release but yes, why don't we talk about it? It's odd, isn't it?

Well, I don't think it is odd because at one point in history, the wise women were revered in communities and people would go to the wise woman, for her remedies, for her counsel, for healing. The patriarchy didn't tolerate that. They perceived our power and potency as a threat to their order, so we were burned at the stake. We were silenced, literally, we were silenced.

We feel that in our bones so, it comes as no surprise to me that we haven't for so very long, talked about these things, because we feel it at a cellular level, at soul level, we feel it.

Yes, that sense of perhaps persecution, it's not okay. Between ourselves, we don't sit there and discuss these things with our peers. We use sort of code words.

Well yes, because we were also taught to mistrust each other as women. We were taught to be competitive and to mistrust and to bitch about each other.

Yeah, you're right.

You know, it's a big thing for us to open our mouths and our throat chakra and our heart and our womb and say, 'Actually, this is my experience. This is how I feel about it.' And this is what I want to reclaim.

Yeah. There's quite a bit of religion stuff, is it the old Orthodox Jewish faith that say we are unclean when we bleed and you weren't allowed in the kitchen?

I think there's some other religions that don't allow women in the kitchen to prepare food because you're unclean in your blood time.

Yes, so it's not surprising really, is it? And it's not surprising that we find it difficult to talk about it with our partners, because they have also grown up with the patriarchy and it's also damaged them. It's difficult for them to make sense of it and to have the conversation and to broach the conversation

That's all made me think and I remember saying to my husband, when we were much younger, "We haven't made love for a whole week, is that wrong?"

We were never a couple who were making love all the time. There was a lot of pressure that everybody had to be having sex all the time or there was something wrong with you. I have listened to clients, so many people, within my work, young people in relationships. They are not making love, they are not having intercourse. They have a sexless marriage. It wasn't to begin with. And even I think, 'Whoa, that's not right.' That's my judgment. I've got to remove that one out because then I realise, that's my stuff – the judgment that if you're young, you've got to be doing it.

Yes, I find the judgments, my own included, very interesting. Even in the spiritual world, I listen to podcasts where people say as we get older it's really important to maintain a sex life. And I think, well, hang on a second, let's stop and have a conversation about this. I don't find another person telling me that this is how I should be feeling, this is what I should be doing, is very enlightened. I think it may help all of us to just take a breath and really talk about this. Let us explore this.

Totally. Otherwise, we all start feeling guilty that we're not. It shouldn't be a pressure on us. Everyone is different. Some people will be having amazing sexual relationships with their partners till they're in their eighties, nineties. Some people will not. I don't think there's any right or wrong with it. It's about how the relationship is and I think that for me, it's been a hard thing to tell my husband because I don't want him to think I don't fancy him. But it's my journey. I think this is important what we've discussed today. It's a tough one.

Thank you. Thank you for your honesty and your openness with that.

Okay. So, how do you feel about being a woman now that you are a Crone? I mean, I think you have spoken a fair bit about that. Is there anything else that you want to add?

It's so funny but I don't like the word Crone. I still struggle with Crone. It sounds really ugly sometimes. Just horrible.

Do you know what Crone means?

No, I'm not sure I do. What does it mean?

A wise woman, a Crone is a wise woman. It is a word that people retract from because it's become a word that means old, ugly, no longer a valid woman. The patriarchy has taken the word and used it as an insult, a derogatory word, to diminish women, to take our power and potency. Again, it is unsurprising that we retract when we hear the word Crone, that we exclaim, 'Oh no, I'm not that. I don't want to be that.' And actually, we are denying the very thing we become, a wise, potent powerful woman.

Crone means wise woman!

Oh, that's strong conditioning, isn't it? Conditioning that we are not what we are. What comes in when I hear Crone is that picture of the witch with a great big nose and warts and is not beautiful. So, that's my conditioning, I put my hands up to it!

It's interesting connecting with words. The wise woman. Yes. How does it feel to be a Crone? It's good. Actually, it's good, I'm okay. I thought, when I look back, that I would know everything. I realise I went through exactly what I needed to, to have this confidence.

And I am slowing down. COVID of course has slowed us down even more. And that is one of the blessings in this time, slowing down and coming back to self. It's given me that opportunity. Well, the whole world needs it. The planet needs it, we all need it. For me personally, what I'm doing now is I'm having to slow that energy down. I can now really know when I'm trying to do three things at once. I can do some of it tomorrow! I've started to really try and not overdo things because I still get overwhelmed.

How does that show up for you?

What has changed is, I do get overwhelmed when I have too much to do. I used to burn energy off and get off on being really busy. Now I go, 'Oh gosh,' I can do this or that tomorrow. I have to find balance on that because I could just become reclusive. I think, 'Oh no,' I don't want to be doing anything, but you know, I need to connect. I need to be out there. I need to be doing whatever I need to do and working. And so, I have to get the balance of not retreating completely, which is part of what my energy is about. I am very happy about being quiet and on my own. I'm not on my own because I have my husband. But you know, just not connecting to the outside world at all is easy for me to slip into. But yeah, it's been good.

It's been a real lesson and I think that's one of the things about getting older. I do get tired more easily. I can't mentally or physically do what I used to do. I remember my cousin telling me about five, six years ago, she said, "Louise, you've just got to slow down! I actually look forward to my little nap in the afternoon."

I was so horrified. I thought, 'Oh, you are getting into your old age far too early.' And I was really judgmental. I was thinking, 'How could you be doing that? You are too young. Shut up.' Now I have got to acknowledge that I *need* to take time out. COVID has really helped on that.

So, physically, mentally I have slowed down a bit. That's what I've noticed, and spiritually connecting. I want to say being wise; I think I have a wisdom and a *trust* and have more confidence in connection to my wisdom. But I still sometimes think I know nothing, as the challenges of the world and the planet and humans, that is actually one thing I thought I would know it all by now!

I love that about being Crone. I know what I know with wisdom and I also know with wisdom, that I know nothing.

Yes. Lovely, wonderful, I love that. Perfect. Yes. Definitely. Great quote! I think that's right. And it's also *admitting* and *acknowledging* that I know nothing. I know everything and I know nothing. And I think that's being mature enough to acknowledge both. And that gives me a confidence. I felt that I knew nothing through my life, and I now know that I *do* know something and what I do know, I have wisdom in. That's lovely. I mean the Crone; she's always been inside us. She's always been there.

I wonder how much we connect to that wisdom, the Soul part, throughout our life – the child; the baby? I think in my twenties I kind of lost it. I kind of lost that connection and that wisdom as I just hurtled my way through the world. It was coming into my thirties that I started to get my psychic information. I did Reiki and I suddenly started connecting back to that. It's wonderful to see the pattern. I'm going to draw that actually. I'm going to do it as a timeline for myself, sort of the worldly and the spiritual and just see where I'm at. I'll do that after this and see what I'll tune in to, see what I feel instinctively.

I love that idea Louise, drawing a timeline to connect to your pathways.

So, we're coming to the end, you spoke about your journey with your ovaries at the beginning of this. Is there anything that you want to add about your relationship with your womb and your yoni?

Mmm, that's interesting. About a year ago, I started connecting to the moon and the stars, the moon very strongly. I have never really done that before. I'm really interested in nature and plants and trees, the sun, being outside. I am really connected to nature.

But the moon is really interesting.

And I think that was to connect back to my womb really because I don't have the cycles anymore. I guess I don't feel so connected to that aspect. What do I feel?

I feel perhaps on the spiritual, Soul level I'm connected. But the physical aspect? Do I need it anymore as I come through into old age and toward death, do I need that physical connection? I think we must need a physical connection to *every* part of us. Perhaps our breasts are there to remind us of the connection to our female aspect once our cycle is gone?

That's fascinating that you say that. The focus of my work has been womb. That was my initiation, being diagnosed with a uterine fibroid. In the past few months, well, actually the sensations I have been having in my breast have been for over a year, so I've been looking at that, saying, 'Okay, so this voice has shifted from womb to breast'. I'm really fascinated by that and that's what I'm sitting with and the not knowing. There's definitely something around that though. Our breasts are about nourishment and the mother. It's interesting to move from a womb focus to a breast focus.

Perhaps it's that feminine aspect of ourselves? Oh, I love that. I get cold chills around my chest when something's really coming in, either for myself or somebody else. I got cold chills as you said that about the breast – that's an interesting confirmation for you, an affirmation in some way? Like looking to see what your hot flushes are telling you.

I love that Louise, beautiful. I think that's a lovely place to stop. A piece for us both to take time and reflect on. What are our breasts communicating to us?

Reflective Questions

What resonated with you from Louise's story?

What insights have you gleaned?

What is your biggest takeaway?

SHARIE

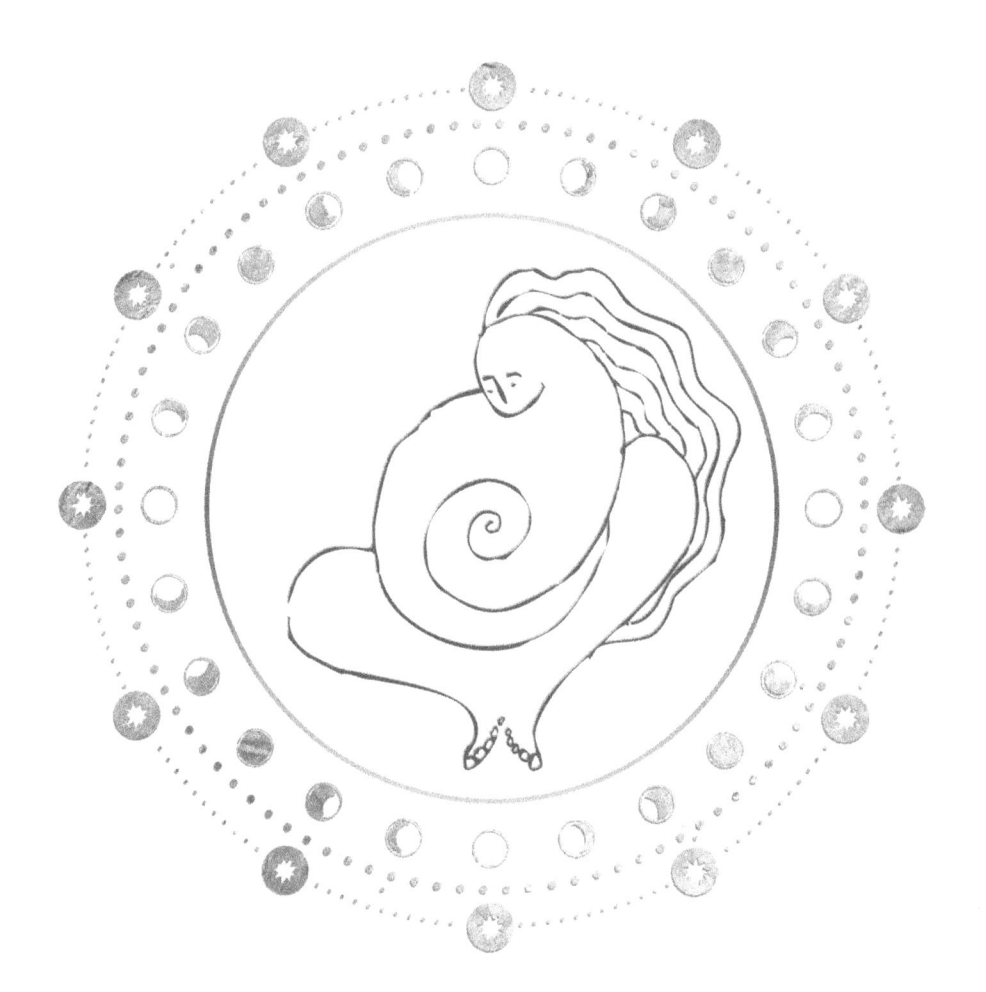

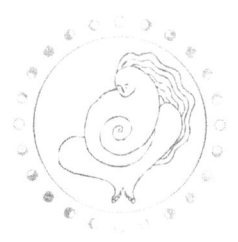

What have you been told, taught and shown about what it is to be a woman?

I grew up in a predominantly matriarchal house, but the needs of the men always came first. My dad was a miner. He would come in after work covered in the black soot of the coal, fall asleep upright with a cup of tea in his hand and a cigarette still burning. The whole energy was, strong women make sure their men are happy, then they get peace.

A core part of me always thought there was something wrong with this. It wasn't a happy home I lived in; there was no space given to independent thought. There were major issues and they brought out the rebel in me. Although we were open and caring and loved each other, it was always about women putting others before themselves.

How old were you when you were first conscious of these attitudes and behaviours and wanting to rebel against them?

I would say when I was about eight; when I was going to other people's houses and seeing their families were different. Certainly, seeing how other mothers interacted with their daughters on a healthy level, which wasn't happening in my home.

I think I always had a sense of the deep power of women together. I would see my grandmother holding seances in the parlour. I would sit there and listen and watch. I'd sneak out of bed and sit on the bottom of the stairs to hear what was going on. Not just of the seances but listening to my parents talking too. The message was always about keeping the men happy. I thought from a very early age, 'That's not right.' My mother wasn't subservient all of the time, but she was always pre-empting, getting the tea ready, whatever it was.

I remember everyone talking about Christmas being this wonderful time of holiday. But we never got to see my mum; she was always out in the kitchen. The main energy of the family was running around like a blue arse fly. I made it a thing with my children from an early age that everything would be done by Christmas Eve, then we would all snuggle up and enjoy Christmas from three o'clock. I was able to sit and enjoy the excitement with my children. I was breaking the pattern; this is what I'm doing. I don't get the attitude of, to be a nurturer you also have to suffer, 'a woman's work is never done' perspective. We can choose, where, when, how, what we are doing. That's how it should be.

You've spoken a little already about how those experiences impacted on you as you transitioned from girl to woman. Is there more you'd like to share?

Seeing other women in my family in abusive relationships, I could see it wasn't working for them! Walking on eggshells, hoping for love and tenderness and support wasn't working; they were running for cover. I witnessed male aggression from a very young age. You can bring them the moon, then the moon is the wrong colour and you still get battered. Subservience isn't love, it certainly isn't respect; it doesn't work.

What are your memories of your menarche, your first bleed?

I was fourteen years old, a late starter and my bleed happened when I was an Air Cadet on the Remembrance Sunday March. That's when I first bled, so I can time it down to the actual day. We finished the march, I went into the Royal British Legion toilet and I thought, 'Okay, it's happened then!' I'd witnessed it with other girls in school who'd started and were talking about buying tampons and it all looked kind of cool. My grandmother (who brought me up) never gave me the sit-down talk beforehand. I gathered the information from other girls, a bit from my biological mum. So, I was in the toilet and I knew I had to do something, so I just wadded up the toilet paper and made myself as comfortable as I could. I remember I had a lemonade! I remember thinking, 'Well, this is what's supposed to happen.' It was late happening, according to all the other girls, which I used to doubt whether it was or wasn't. I was aware of the shift in energy in the other girls when they started to bleed. It was an energy of knowing, 'I now have the ability to make a life.' Every month, that ability to create life, blood is life, blood is power.

Did you feel that at that time of being fourteen or is it something that came to you later in life?

I felt it at the time – I was a strange old kid. I was an old Soul. I was very much a loner. It was only when I went to camp with the other girls in the Air Cadet that I felt that camaraderie. Because of my family, I had a few friends but not a big gang. Most of my experience at school was of being bullied because I was different. People saw me as weird and strange and because of my family, different. But I was someone who thought, 'I'm not changing. You can pick on me and bully me but I'm not changing.'

In that moment, my first bleed, I felt 'Okay, I've *become*.' That's so powerful for a fourteen-year-old to experience.

So, can you tell me more about your grandmother?

Yes. I was adopted and brought up by my grandmother.

And she hadn't talked to you about starting your period?

No. When I got home that day, I told her what had happened and she gave me one of her sanitary towels. They were those big old things in those days. Do you remember them?

Yes, I know what you're going say!

Yeah, they were like mattresses, that's what I called them. I can remember making a bed for my Barbie doll out of one of them.

I used those mattresses until we went into town and into the new Boots and I could pick what I wanted myself. My grandmother was upset because she'd bought me these big plastic knickers. I thought I had to wear them instead of my ordinary knickers but they were for wearing on the outside of your knickers. So, I had stuff to sort out with her. I think I remember her telling me I'd bleed every month. She didn't say anything about sex or boys, which you'd think would be in the forefront of her mind because when I was born, my mother was fourteen. It was a big story with lots of extenuating angles to it.

I think I'd been menstruating for about six months when I met an older boy. He was eighteen – there were lots of warnings. I conceived a child but I didn't carry the child to term. I had a miscarriage. It was an early loss; I remember it looked like a little golden marble with a little pink rosebud centre. That was it. I stood there panicking and the only thing I knew what to do in the end was flush it.

Had you known you were pregnant?

Yes.

Had you told anyone else?

Just the partner I was with. He panicked and, in his panic, he decided to hit me to make sure things wouldn't survive. And I thought, he had hit me hard. A couple of weeks later it passed, I lost it. I think I was about eight, nine weeks pregnant. I don't know if there was anything merciful in what happened actually. It was a massive thing.

My journey into being a woman came from my grandmother saying they (men) own everything you've got. I thought, 'Not my body, you don't.' My brothers escaped from the house, they got a partner, married, left the house. I thought deep in my subconscious, the one thing that you can't have of mine, is if I have a little one. I do own that; I think it was rumbling in the background. When I was sixteen, I conceived again and married. By the time I was nineteen I had two children. I felt, this is *my* body – you don't own it and having children is what I can do, what I can own. You can't have them.

Who can't have them?

My grandmother. I had a mindset of, 'I'll show you who owns me.' It was the only control I had.

When you became pregnant at fourteen, did you know that was the age your mother had you?

I don't think I did quite at that point. It only came out in later years that she'd had me. She had nearly died giving birth – she haemorrhaged. She carried me as an unmarried mother to be. I was due to be adopted out of the family but my grandmother put a stop to it and adopted me to keep me in the family. When my mum got to about sixteen, she couldn't take the awful life she had and she left. She thought they would follow her and give me back to her. But they didn't. She threatened them to take good care of me. She created a new life in England.

When I was seven, my grandparents legally adopted me. My upbringing was really with my grandparents.

On the one hand, my grandmother was quite ahead of her time. She had a power to her and always to its limit, the mother rules, to a point. The boundaries were set by the men.

So how have those experiences shaped your life as a woman?

It's been a big journey because in many ways there have been parallels to my mother in my life. I had a different resilience to her. I had the belief 'no one's allowed to treat me like that'. I found a voice. If I was the kid in the story of the 'King Who's Got No Clothes', I'd be the one in the crowd saying loud and clear 'That king is naked!' I was the one who came out and said 'NO. ENOUGH'.

This was when you had transitioned into woman?

Yes. I'd fallen into the hands of someone quite abusive. When I got to about nineteen, I said, 'Enough.' This pattern is not going to repeat itself. My daughter is not going to learn this pattern. I drew a line. I broke a line of love and abuse that are supposed go hand in hand. They don't. I left. I got out. It made me a fighter.

Maybe it was my inner little shaman that was always growing and kicking, feeling and sensing. All my guides who would come and save me, showing me I had to take my major identity with them. It was in the later years that I knew I had to heal or I would continue to carry cellular memory of the abuse pattern. The experience gave me fight and it gave me resilience. I was the first person in the family to say, 'No.' I am the only woman in my family to divorce. To divorce the abusive man.

You've put a stop to that cycle of abuse?

Yes. As much as I can. I can't stop my daughter making her own choices. My granddaughter, she's a naughty little bugger, she's sixteen. There are things trickling down, things she doesn't understand about certain aspects and I say, 'I can tell you but I think you're too young;' and she asks 'What's age got to do with it?' I tell her she can know the age-appropriate stuff! I've told her, 'If you're with someone and it *feels* wrong, then it *is* wrong. You watch for red flags and you're out. Once you see it, you don't hold onto it, you're out, goodbye.'

These are the messages you're giving to your granddaughter?

Oh God, yeah.

Switching back to the first bleed, not being given any information, the strong memory of when it happened as a Cadet. Did that impact at all on your menopausal experience?

Yeah, I think that the bleeding stopping was a blessing. I saw it as holding my power which was a blessing too. I'd had a miscarriage and I got sterilised at twenty-nine. I had about thirteen miscarriages. Even though I got sterilised, I think I would have loved another child. At a cellular level I thought, 'Oh well, there could be a blistering miracle and I'll have a child.' I know that's a load of crap but when the Menopause came, it allowed the closure. It brought a closure that brought peace. The first bleed was about knowing I had a power, something to control. The journey of my fertility wasn't always kind, wasn't always easy.

I had endometriosis which was quite viscous; I had miscarriages. So, when the Menopause came, I was, 'Oh thank God!' I didn't think I was going to be any less of a woman, I thought, 'Okay, I'm going to be a different woman.' I came into it with a sense of grief and peace; I landed. I found Miranda Gray and the blessing of treating my cycle in the way she teaches. I made peace with my body through the Womb Blessings, the work of Miranda, through the journey of initiating into becoming a Moon Mother together. So, when the Menopause arrived, I was, 'Yeah, bring it on.'

I'm waiting for my hair to turn lovely and white and sparkly! I did dye my hair blonde but men kept rushing to open doors for me, thinking there'd be someone young! I had a blonde moment but I didn't like it. I thought, I'm white, not blonde. Who I am is bugger all to do with the colour of my hair. I have a raw, elemental earth energy that has called me to colour my hair amethyst, my birth stone.

It sounds like you're having fun with it.

Yeah. I feel like (throws arms up in the air), 'Helloooo Menopause, I LOVE you!'

Did you know what to expect? Had you been given any information?

Yes, I tended to have older women friends who taught me about healthy eating, nourishment and the Menopause. I had a friend who had quite a journey through Menopause. She'd tell me about the struggles she had; I thought, 'Oh dear God.' But when I started having those experiences, I felt annoyed with myself that I hadn't known more so I could have been more supportive to that friend. Once you're in those shoes, I thought, 'Holy Bugger! If anyone had told me!'

The fridge would ring because I'd put my phone in there, not knowing I had. Even recently, it's been about two years now since I stopped bleeding, I started working in a café. Memory is pretty handy working in a café! But, oh dear I had brain fog.

I did think it could be gentle or it might not. If it's not, I thought I'd use plant allies to help me. That's one of the things my friend taught me early on in her journey through the Menopause. She had tried HRT for a short time but then looked at the risks of taking it and came off it pretty sharpish. The main thing she realised was that HRT wouldn't get her through it and then be free of it.

I thought there is too much risk involved with taking HRT. We've got cancer running through the women in my family, so I have a five percent more risk than other women to start with. So, I never even considered it. I went straight to the world of plant allies and *listening* to my body. If my mind was in a scramble, I'd sit down and take a rest.

So, that sounds like you really brought in the element of honouring your body, knowing when you needed to stop and rest. Is that what you did?

Yes, I actually became self-employed in order to do that. I came out of working in the Care sector, because my brain fog didn't allow me to think straight. And my heart space changed, I didn't like what I saw around me, how people were being treated. And my bleeding at that point was so severe, I was losing about half a pint in two days. I used a moon cup and a pad and I was still soaked. I looked at my moon cup as a chalice that was holding my blood, the last magic of my body. There was a little bit of prolapse too which I treated homoeopathically.

So, when the Menopause really kicked in, I used sage, rest. There were moments when I had what I called a fuddled head and I did feel exasperated. I was a woman who had got on a plane on her own and flew to stay in Australia for six weeks. When I was menopausal, I went to the supermarket. There was a bunch of kids yelling and screaming. I couldn't stand the disruption, so I got a bunch of bananas, no other provisions, and went home. I couldn't handle the energy in that moment. I remember my friend describing such moments, which was a comfort to know.

I had books and connecting with sisterhood in Circle and it felt okay. The Menopause wasn't fun to go through but I realise I wasn't 'losing my marbles.'

Can you expand on those experiences. Were there things you particularly liked about being menopausal?

I had never known how to let anything go over my head. I was an overthinker. When the Menopause started kicking in, I developed a different attitude. I was someone who had been trained into thinking I should do everything asked of me. With the Menopause I have learnt to say, 'No!' I'm fine with upsetting people if they don't get what they want from me. It may sound like I'm being nasty, but it's not that. I discovered I had the ability to not turn myself inside out for someone else. And, when someone treated me badly, I told them to 'sod off.' For someone like me who was indoctrinated by my grandmother to be a 'good girl,' to serve others, put them before yourself for your whole life, I am still Mother, but I do it now to *my* rhythm.

So, would you say you are choosing when to give and when not to give, setting your boundaries?

Oh yes. Give me boundaries, I love the boundaries. When I'm putting out food now, I put the best potato on *my* plate! That juicy bit of meat there, that's going on *my* plate! Now I am a woman who has her plate full first, then I'll do your plate.

Were there any aspects of the Menopause you really didn't like?

Hot flushes – I had internal central heating. I still do get them now and again. One of the ways I managed the Menopause was to work from home. I could control my environment and not be so physical. Now I'm working in a café, a physical environment, the hot flushes have come back. Worst of all though, the brain fog came back too. I hit the ground running at the café. I was put in the kitchen and asked to supervise. By the second week, the flushes and brain fog returned and they thought, 'What the hell is going on with her?'

To compound it, my iron levels dropped. The orders coming into the kitchen may as well have been written in alien. It was like having Alzheimer's; it was terrifying. I was thinking, 'Please be the Menopause causing this.' I didn't want it to be early dementia.

Would you say then that you have identified for yourself that putting yourself in stressful situations has caused the return of those symptoms you describe?

Yes. It's a very physical job. I found the brain fog cruel because I didn't feel like me. I became a spiralling fool; I couldn't do my job properly. But my boss persevered and told me to slow down. I've been taking iron tablets and doing more strategic things to ground myself. I use my crystals, take Rescue Remedy (Bach Flower Remedy). That really helps with my anxiety. When anxiety kicks in, everything else goes to hell. And that is definitely from being menopausal. I wasn't a person who ever felt lonely. I've loved my own company all my life. I told a friend I started to have these feelings; I don't think it was depression but my friend said, 'You're lonely. What you're describing is loneliness.' I found that really hard, I'd rather be depressed than lonely. I was really angry; I don't do lonely.

Do you think that was triggering rage?

Yes, Menopause changed how I responded to stuff. No more gentle patience with bullshit.

Would you say the rage was a part of a healing process?

Oh yes, it was like fireworks in my aura. I could feel it in my aura, a tingling and a boomf, boomf! And it felt like, 'Yeah! Come on, enough already!'

Did it feel like you were letting go of stuff?

Yes, and I enjoyed it. I had always been taught that no-one around me should ever feel bad. Now, I say, 'You can choose how you want to feel, but I'm not having it.' I had a voice.

I gave myself permission to be me.

I stopped apologising. The whole tiptoeing around people no longer worked for me. I was very charged; it was like having boils lanced, such a relief. All the venom was released.

That's a great analogy.

Second interview one year later

Goodness, a year has passed so quickly! I'm excited to complete your Menopause wisdom interview. And the first question is, what do you see when you look in the mirror?

The good thing about me is I have never been, 'Oh my god I can't stand my body,' or 'I've got to diet.' I don't do dieting. I've never done it. I've watched my diet because of kidney stones and that's as far as it got. I watched my diet because of breast cysts and that was as bad as it got. I've never been, 'Oh my god,' I can't look at myself in the mirror.'

I think especially when you're menopausal, you get more cravings, like when you are a pregnant woman, that's what I found. So, when I look in the mirror, I'm like, 'This is it,' and, 'This is all me.'

It's quite interesting really, because I would say that they might not class me as obese, but I was like a comfortable size sixteen, eighteen. And God knows what sizes I was really, because with gluten intolerance, I could be fourteen in the morning and a twenty by the night. So, yeah, I've never thought, 'Oh I can't look in the mirror,' but I never spent a lot of time looking anyway – unless it was just to make sure everything was set before I went out the door, checking my tights weren't hanging over the back of my jeans.

But I have started getting back into my femininity now because I did lose some weight. I did have quite a belly; I had quite an overhang. So, I hadn't really seen much below my hips for a while. I've lost a bit of weight now. I'm down to twelve stone again, so I've sort of been like, 'Oh hello,' and I am like, 'Well, god when did my pubes turn white?' I thought my partner would have said something. That was quite funny really. But I mostly just like who I am because there are bigger things you can feel miserable about. If I lost an arm or a leg, I think I would still be, 'Well, you know, you are what you are.'

I hear what you have said about your physical being and how you feel about that. What if you go beyond the physical, if you were to look deeply into your own eyes, what do you see?

I think, when I vision myself, I do feel more crowned. I do still have a lot of Menopause symptoms – I've got the spots of a teenager. I do still have quite a few symptoms, even though I am post-menopausal. I bled for a spell – it still rises to bite me in the ass every now and again. But I do see myself as crowned and empowered. If I were to really look deep, if I were to vision myself, I want my hair to turn fully sparkly white.

It hasn't gone white yet, so I say, 'Stuff it,' and I turned it purple! But yeah, I see myself as empowered at this time, especially with the choice that I made about my relationship with my partner. Now I'm *this* person, I give my opinion with confidence, not apologising. I'm not about to agree with you if I don't. I guess I'm owning my own place in the world.

I'm careful with it because I'm very aware of the 'beast' inside. I ask myself, 'Right where is me? Where is the beast?' I think that's something I said to my partner. That's how I made my choice because that's part of where I am at right now. I was asking, 'What was me, what was us?' And I guess in a way, I needed to make sure what was *not* related to being menopausal. But the choice I made further on *was* to do with the Menopause. It made me own the importance of what I did.

Do you think that is the wisdom of being Crone? To be able to distinguish?

What I did, I didn't do it from the Menopause. I did it from feeling bloody wretched, feeling totally wretched and despondent. When I was getting in a good space, I was like, 'Don't bring me down.'

I'm still working on it a lot. I would say I'm more on the Crone side now but there are still things, like the hormones, that are left. No, I have my space; I'm knowing my right to my space in this world whether I'm good, whether I'm bad and that's it.

What are your feelings about sex and your sexuality now that you are post-menopausal? If you can think about how that has or hasn't changed throughout your whole Menopause experience and how that relates to your decision to end your relationship.

I think when I was doing it, it was like being a teenager again. I would have moments where I would suddenly just want to eat the person alive, but then if he touched me, everything he did was wrong.

I felt like, don't do this, that's wrong. It was like part of myself that I really knew well became quite alien. Nothing felt the same and at that point where I needed more support, he would push my button, and bang, done. It was like learning to rewire, I had to learn that my body was rewiring itself. And I think because I was someone that had a lot of negative experiences through my life and had managed to compartmentalise them to be resilient, my own sexuality was still there. There was still pleasure and power that was my own. So, to have the Menopause coming in and screwing around with that, made it at times feel quite good. I was like, 'Well, this is just me now.'

Do you feel that there was any grief around that loss of what had been familiar to you?

Yes. I think that is a good way of putting it, yeah, I would say grief. Because I was fierce. I was passionate. I was wicked as sin. I was like, 'I am woman!' And then it was like, 'I can't be arsed with this anymore.'

At moments it has started to get extraordinarily strong, very recently, this last month; I don't know if it's in connection with taking my power back in other ways, but I am owning my body more. I think it's since I went out to work in the café. That created a change because of how I was being seen by others. Suddenly, I have people coming in and being cheeky and flirting with me and I'm thinking, 'I have no idea how to respond to this.' There was somebody that sort of threw it out there that he liked me and that started making me see myself in a whole different way. I wasn't interested in returning it, but it was like, 'Oh wow, okay I am a girl.' I mean it was part of the process of looking at all of me, just as me, who I am as a woman, what I want, what I deserve.

Did you experience some of those changes when you were in your relationship with your partner?

Yeah.

How was that for you in terms of the relationship? Were you able to stand in your authority?

I think what happened in the relationship is, it was circling the drain. I had very frank open conversations with him.

Then all sorts of things were dropping in and I think as my body was starting to reset itself and the sexuality and the sensuality was coming back, I thought, 'This is coming back and it's not going to be appreciated.' There's no home for this with him, and I didn't particularly want to do it with anyone else either. But I was like, hang on, I'm coming back to life and I'd been with him for eleven years, there should be a home for this to thrive back into and there isn't. When that was done, we split up. And I thought I'd rather enjoy me again, you know?

Yes, I do. I think this is the stuff that we don't talk about and yet it feels so important. So, yes, I really honour and appreciate you sharing your experience.

Okay. So, at this stage in your life, do you feel that you are connected to your womb and yoni?

Oh god, yeah. Story of my life, it came slowly. But yes, I am connected to my womb and yoni, on a sensual level and a spiritual level. I love to dance. When I dance it's from my womb.

As much as I have a lot of bravado, I'm not actually a big show off but I was out on the dance floor recently and I owned it! I found my Goddess within. Oh my god! That night I was owning all of me and I was totally a Goddess. My hair was flowing, I was in flow.

How did that make you feel?

I felt like the Goddess in the ring. I was totally like, this is me. I danced it all out. And I'm in a choir now, and even though we can't be together (due to Covid restrictions) when I'm practicing, it's from my womb, my voice, my groove, it's from my womb, beautiful. I think it's wonderful because I'm also at peace about the bleeding; that power was mine, I'm like, 'Wow'!

I've got this power source that is constantly renewing itself. It's there, it's an internal cycle.

Since the blood has stopped?

Yeah. This is an energy that built up and it goes nowhere, so I can think, 'Right, what do I want? Where am I? What will I do with this energy today? What magic will we be doing together today?'

That's gorgeous, I love that.

So how do you feel about being a woman now that you are, post-

menopausal, a Crone? Is there anything else you want to say?

Yeah, I think there is a sense of arriving. I can be a woman now and I don't have to worry about being a woman. Because I made peace with my cycle when it ended. Before the bleeding stopped, it was cruel. I was losing something like half a pint in two days.

I made peace with it through the work of Miranda Gray. I just love the fact that I can just plan my life now and be organised. I don't have to think of the, 'What ifs?' and the chaos that could happen.

I am free to go and dance in the rain as much as I damn well want. I am free to use my body.

And I wasn't put on this earth just to bring pleasure for men or children.

I am all woman, all for me now.

I think as well, what the Menopause has done for me, is it helped me heal. There's been a lot of closure. It's like, that door closed and I'm arriving as my own woman. I'm not my mothers.

Beautiful, thank you Sharie. I love the magic you have in your cauldron. Such gems for other woman to connect with.

Yeah, it's like an arrival.

That resonates for me – the healing that arrives with Menopause is so powerful.

I am so thankful that you have invited me to do this. It's been lovely, a privilege too. Making a change for our daughters and our sisters. And letting people know to be *kind* to women who are going through the Menopause. I've started to talk to younger women about the Menopause. They are curious. The more you're prepared, the less fear there is.

Reflective Questions

What resonated with you from Sharie's story?

What insights have you gleaned?

What is your biggest takeaway?

SITALI

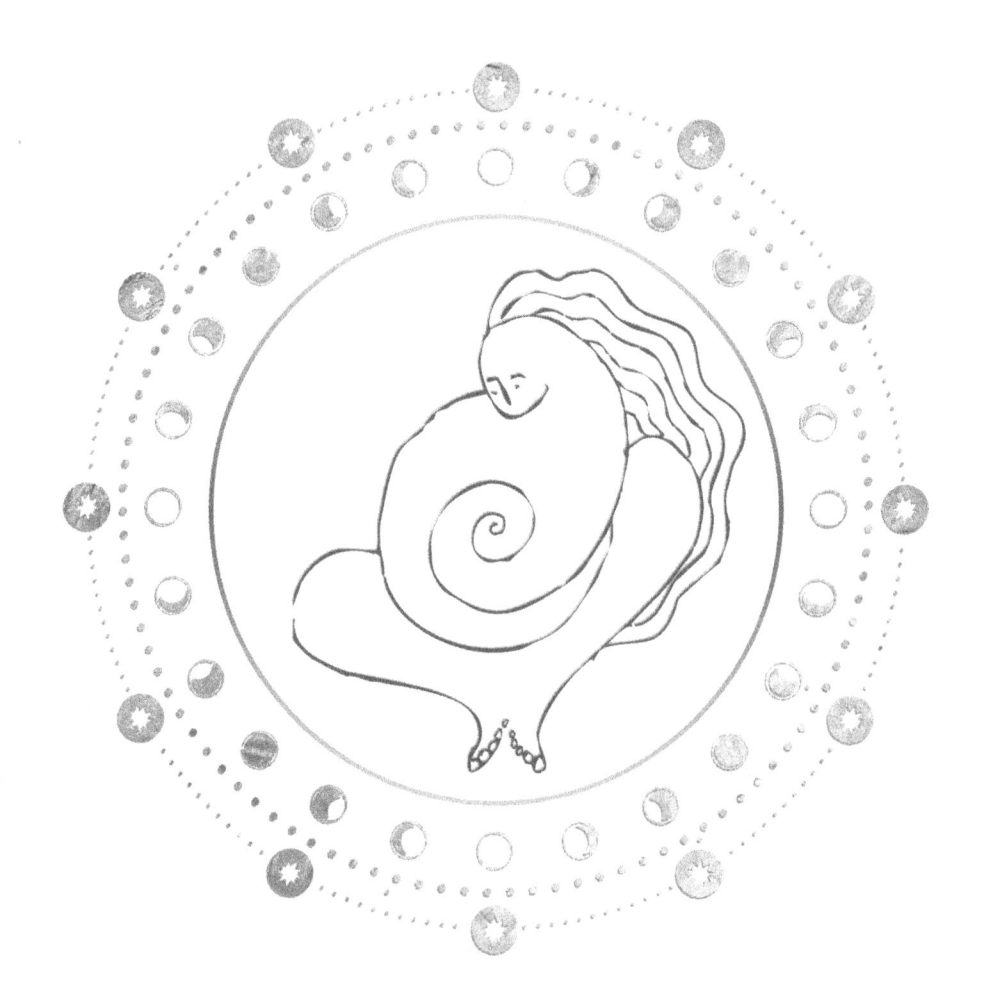

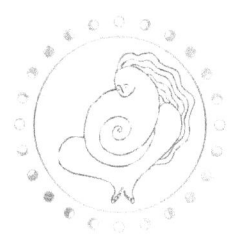

What have you been told or taught about what it is to be a woman? Think back to the first messages you were given from your mother, father, friends, media.

I wasn't aware of any gender differences at all when I was a child. My mother was not there, my father was both father and mother figure in my life, very protective. I had older siblings, one in particular who was at home, the much older one was away working in a different city. The second older female figure that formed a mother figure in the house, she was a bit of a tomboy in herself, so she never really restricted us or anything like that. But occasionally when the first born would come and visit, she was very feminine in herself, very strict I suppose in how she would expect us to sit as a woman or a girl, with our legs crossed, making us aware of our bodies. Apart from that there just wasn't any differentiation gender ways. I was completely unaware of being female. Although now, looking back and hearing stories later on as an adult, I am aware of it now. But as a child, no. It was unusual for an African child, from a tribal point of view.

Did this change for you as you transitioned from being a teenager to a young woman?

The transition happened for me within the last decade, the real transitioning that I was aware of. Before that, no. Now that I've transitioned, I'm more aware of what has actually been going on.

When I started my periods, I wasn't aware. But what I was made aware of when I started my period was that I was fortunate, because in our tribe, when a woman transitions, when the menstrual cycle kicks in, they have a ritual. It's not a very embracing one. It's like a training thing where you are pinched; you are told to sit properly, you are told to be a home keeper as your role as woman. And there were many other things that I don't know about, because our father protected us from it. He only protected us because we were a family of eight, four of each. The first two women went through it, but the last two didn't, including me.

What I realise now is that my mum is a feminist at heart – stronger – and so she had those strengths. She never encouraged us to be female and fight for us. She believed in us defining ourselves, I think. Looking at her journey, when she came back to Zambia, having studied in the UK, she had a big battle because she was told, quite rightly, that you can have all the education you like in the UK. But here in Zambia, and as a woman, you have a low standing. So that became apparent to me. It's been reading books on feminism, encouraging me to look at materials, articles, those kinds of things. And also, I guess, as my daughter, with her menstrual cycle and thankfully the retreat you held, that my husband Paul got me to go to, was the real eye opener for me. It helped me to realise who I am in the present, as a female. The body that we're carrying, that our cycle, our period is not a curse, it's a part to embrace. It's those aspects from your input, which you've been a very strong figure in my life, even from the moment we met, with my daughter and everything.

Thank you. It's an honour to be told that Sitali.

Interestingly, yesterday I was at a do, a Christmas do. One of my bosses, (female) she came over to talk to me about something; and she was looking at me and looking at my phone. I was looking at the menstrual cycle app, and she kind of shrieked, 'What are you looking at that for!

I said, 'Sally, when you started your periods, were you aware of your cycle, and how did it all happen for you?'

She said, 'I just told my mum. I didn't actually have any education – I just told my mum, 'Mum I'm on heat,' and then she got me some pads'.

I love that you responded with a question to invite her to reflect on her own experience. If we have those conversations with other women, to educate and support each other through our transitions, we start to claim the potency of our menstrual cycle and then we can move into Menopause with cyclical knowledge, with growing wisdom.

So, let's talk about your first bleed, can you remember when you started menstruating and what was it like for you?

The whole gender thing although it wasn't instilled in us, the differences, from a gender point of view, there was no education, no science class. I had older women in my life, because I was the youngest sister, but I never saw any pads. I think my older sister started after me probably, my much older one's though, they had their cycles and I never came across any pads or anything, really.

I went to the bathroom, and realised there was blood and told my older female figure, my mother figure in the family, my sister, and she said, "Oh, go and use a pad. This is how you use it."

I was scared, because we didn't have showers, only a bath tub, we have more bath tubs in Zambia than showers. I was worrying about getting in the bath tub and if it was going to hurt like an open wound. That's all that comes to mind.

Wow, that's powerful. Was there any conversation between you and your older sister about being scared?

No, nothing like, 'This is going to happen,' or 'This is going to come on a monthly basis,' nothing about how you go about it. I was still in primary school, and at school we didn't talk about it.

How did you manage your cycle? What was it like for you? Was it an easy cycle? Do you recall any pain, or changes in emotions? Did you have any consciousness about what was happening?

No, I had no consciousness. I was talking to my sister when my daughter was experiencing bad cramps with her cycle and she said, "Oh yeah, you used to have really terrible cramps!"

I don't remember I ever did, so I was completely unaware. It just didn't register, no resentment, nothing.

So how has that experience impacted on you as you became a more mature woman, moving into your creative, mother phase, of life? That time in which we develop our creative energy, as a mother, our career, our home? Do you feel the experience has impacted on this next phase of your life?

I guess so, I think a lot of my childhood was quite pain stricken. A lot of it I've blanked out, which is maybe why I can't remember so much. Things like how I felt, because there's been a lot of pain. My way of dealing with pain in the past is just to sweep it under the carpet and get on with it. Not having a mother was a big part and the way I've dealt with that was to try and find somebody. I had my older sister and one of our helpers, who was resident; and my uncles' wives hung around our home, but there were never really discussions about being a woman, and being what we call *Mwalanjo* – that's a fruitful woman – our cycle, that discussion wasn't had. And because my mother wasn't there, it's just been blanketed over.

Tell me a little bit about where you think you are in relation to Menopause? Do you feel you have stepped onto that pathway yet or do you feel you are approaching it?

The past two years, mostly last year, I first really noticed changes when I started to wake up and the bed would be soaked in sweat, saturated. Being a hospital person, and someone who is in denial maybe, at one point I thought maybe I should make an appointment with my GP. Maybe I am running a fever, because the sweating wasn't going away.

The past six months, it hasn't happened so much. But last year it was a lot. It was only in conversation with you when you mentioned Menopause, I thought, 'Blimey!' Yes, night sweats, heavier periods, noticing through using my App the regularity of my cycle was changing – the Miranda Gray App you recommended has really helped. It's changed our lives, my daughter's as well.

So, my periods are getting heavier, I'm experiencing stomach cramps which I didn't have before. I've always bumbled along never noticing any pain. I'm realising there are changes, big clots that I never had really. I'm more anxious, I've got lots of anxiety. Looking around for a few materials on Menopause, now I realise these are the changes I am experiencing.

The awareness that you have now and how you're really consciously working with your changes sounds amazing. So, can you say how you are feeling about these changes and your new awareness?

I feel blessed, grateful, and a lot of it is because of you. Because of the energy that you put out, the awareness, the education, the connection. You know, there was a period in my life where I didn't care, I didn't clock when my periods would come. I would realise you know, my period was there, then it was a week ago and I wasn't clocking the dates. I'm resentful because I'm like, 'Oh gosh here's my period again.' But, every time I find myself having those feelings now, I feel, no actually, this is a positive thing. This is something that I should embrace as it's happening. So, in relation to what is going on now, every time I come to those negative feelings, I think I'm more accepting now. I'm opening up to have more knowledge.

You've mentioned night sweats, which I can really relate to, and that your blood is changing, how heavy it is and the clots and the anxiety and again, that resonates for me. So, if I say the word 'rage,' does that resonate at all?

Yes, I have put down rage in my journal. I think the past two or three months I have been raging.

How does that show up for you? In what form does that rage come and when does it come? How do you deal with it?

I try and talk about it with my husband. I think now that I am having some awareness of where I am in terms of my transition, like the mother not being there. She is in Zambia at the moment and I'm thinking, am I going to lose her again? So, that's what the anxiety, the rage is. Sometimes it comes across as, like yesterday I was raging towards a patient, raging in my mind. I was quite abrupt and thinking, 'How dare you!' He, the patient, was asking me where I was born, how many qualifications I've got. If they were all from Zambia, I would be overqualified for this job. I was raging. My answers were very controlled, 'Yes, I was born and brought up in Zambia and I am Zambian.' And, you know, I am free to do anything. I don't need to be raging in my response but it is identity, that's what it is. Because when you are comfortable with who you are, where you are, you don't need to rage and I think it's that.

So, when these things to do with my perception of who I am, where I am from, being comfortable with who I am, then I want to rage if I am anxious. And it's okay because that was the past, it's not now. So, things like that, cause me to have these raging episodes and impatience. Sometimes I feel that I have made those mistakes before. Shouldn't people know that they shouldn't be saying these things?

It's really interesting to hear how your rage is coming in. What the trigger is and how you're dealing with it. I felt that rage was such an important part of the transition on the pathway to becoming Crone, and for me it was very much about understanding what my wounding was.

I was taught that women should not be angry; that we should be good girls and that rage is not acceptable from us. So, when I first started to feel rage, I found it very difficult to find a way to express it. Mine too came out as irritability, but when I understood more about what the rage was, I found practices to allow me to express it and to know that it really was *okay for me to feel and to express that rage. I learnt not to direct it at an individual face to face. I might have been raging about an individual but I would go off and give it to the trees into the valley.*

How do you feel the rage is important to you? Because what I am hearing from you is that it's teaching you, showing you aspects of yourself and the past that need to be looked at and healed?

Yeah. So, I notice the rage comes out when I feel challenged as a mother because of the connection between myself and my daughter, that cord. So, I get rage about that but I have also found that I'm now, a little bit, getting better. Well, not *better* because like you say, it's a process. It's 'fight or flight' and in some instances I purposely choose flight.

So, I run. I exercise and I use that as a way of getting the rage away because I know I can digest things and see things better and process them in my mind when the energy is put somewhere else.

Interestingly, you are the second woman that uses running as a practice.

Did you know what to expect as you began your transition into Menopause? I know a little of this because we had conversations at the retreat. Is there anything else that you want to say about when you started to consciously think, 'I am a woman and at some point, I am going to become menopausal.'

Yes. The retreat was empowering because for the first time ever I was in a circle of women. In terms of the process, the feelings, those things I didn't know and also revisiting the Menopause chapters in your book (*Take of Your Armour*); all of that has been very empowering. The teachings are immense.

Yes, sitting in circle with other women can be such healing medicine.

So, because your mother was absent, I wonder, do you have any recollection of her experience of the Menopause?

No, I think I must have been talking about periods and mentioned in passing, 'Do you need pads or something?'

And she said, "I don't have periods anymore," and that was the end of it.

Last month my sister was visiting and we talked a little bit about Menopause.

She finished her menses when she was 44 years old. She said it was very brief, lots of hot flushes and her periods they just stopped. So, it was a beautiful visit because we were able to catch up on being children. There was also lots of dynamics going on too but intermittently we had little bits about being women.

How did that feel to have those little snippets of conversation?

Liberating, because as a child everything was gated, everything was provided for, never really questioned. There was physical abuse in the house and it all just bumbled along and some stuff is masked because of survival mentally.

But this visit was a visit filled with fruits, amazing fruits, positive, forgiving. And just being able to go back to my mum's. I dropped my sister off at my mum's. We had a drink in the pub, we stayed with my niece and we walked home and then giggling away at one o'clock in the morning. There was nowhere for me to sleep so I slept in the same bed as my sister. I thought, 'Oh wow.' So, we shared the bed together and it took me back to me being her mum as children. I was exhausted because we were giggling away like little kids in the boarding school we went to. Sleeping and waking up and having her holding my hand, hugging my shoulder. It was like being the mother.

Then my brother came to visit. The dynamics were interesting because then three of us were together with *him* being our mum and our mum being left out. She was the spectator but she just let us be. It was interesting!

That made me all tingly and tearful Sitali. That's so beautiful to hear you express how open you are to experiencing what comes up in the dynamics of those different relationships within your family.

Have there been any aspects of your Menopause experience so far that you have disliked?

I think the rage. I haven't liked waking up in cold beds, freezing cold, I don't like that.

And what aspects of it do you like? Can you specify anything you have really so far enjoyed about your menopausal journey?

I like the energy it's bringing, as well the patience, the ability to live and let live more. I love it when I look at my hair, I got the streaks.

It looks gorgeous! I love it. I got the same, like streak sisters.

I love the doors that are being flung open, the connectivity. It's bringing sort of like the ray of light that has always been. And just allowing your gifts to me, for me to embrace being in the company of other women. I love that. Yeah.

Okay, so we both just talked about our grey streaks. When you look in the mirror if you do, because not every woman does, what do you see?

I see my skin is not as elastic and so very young and glowing as it used to be. I see some contours of life and I question sometimes whether they are from frowning. The silver streaks and yeah like patches of oiliness, a bit uneven.

So that's describing the physical manifestation of the changes. How do you feel emotionally about those?

I haven't connected from an emotional point of view. So, I'm not looking and going 'Who is that?' I keep waiting for that moment when I go, 'Oh my goodness, look at you,' I haven't got there yet.

What are your feelings about your sexuality and sex as a menopausal woman?

Interesting one, because my sexuality has always been, my character has always been one of sitting on the fence, always. I think I am attractive to both sexes and attracted as well. Yeah. I feel like…I am fine.

Do you at this point in your life feel connected to your womb energy?

Not as much as I should be, not really no.

When you say 'not as much as you should be' what does that actually mean?

So, I could work better in a connected format with my womb. I can use it because it's there, it's me. I can use it in the peaks, when I'm energetic, hyper – this one I need to tone down. I can work with my womb better but I'm not. That's the most important part about neglecting my womb because at work, when I make arrangements, 'Come and meet with me,' and I'm about to have my period and really, I need to slow down at that point.

You spoke earlier about using running as a practice to focus and clear your mind. Are you at all drawn to creating or following other practices to deepen your connection to your womb? Is that something that you want to do, and if you do, what is stopping you from doing that?

I'm exploring two things I'm doing as a software practice. So, on a Sunday I will wake up early. I'll go for a run – it could be 10k – and then I come home, have a shower and go to church which is around the corner. I learn a lot from that. And I used to do yoga but I haven't in a while. I would love to be connected to my womb. When I looked at Miranda Gray's website you told me about, I couldn't find any Moon Mothers holding a circle here. And you mentioned your monthly connection but at the time I was transitioning with work. But I would love to.

Yes, you could join the monthly Menopause Wisdoms group online.

Yes, it's about connecting with other women. I just need to look into it and just move.

If you go to Miranda's website you can download for free the Full Moon Meditations and register to take part at home. Although you won't be physically in circle with other women, you will be connecting to many thousands who will also be sitting at those times.

Six in the evening or midnight or midday or six in the morning. You can create your own sacred space, create your own altar, have your two bowls. All the instructions are there on the website. Maybe you and Davita could do it together? Experiment with it and have fun with it. Something I definitely have learnt over the years is to have fun with it.

Yes. That sounds good.

So, moving on from your womb connection to my final question which is, do you feel you have a connection with your yoni?

No, not at all. I would be interested, amazing to share and have more awareness.

I put this question in because although I have worked for many years with my womb energy, I hadn't considered until more recently how it would be to connect with my yoni energy, a more complete exploration, I guess. I was really interested to hear other women's experiences.

Perhaps this could be something that we explore as a group of women in the Menopause Wisdoms Circle.

Yes, more awareness and sharing will be amazing.

Great. So, we have all the questions covered, that was beautiful and rich. There's so much for other women to connect with Sitali, thank you.

Thank you. What a gift to do this.

Reflective Questions

What resonated with you from Sitali's story?

What insights have you gleaned?

What is your biggest takeaway?

PEARL

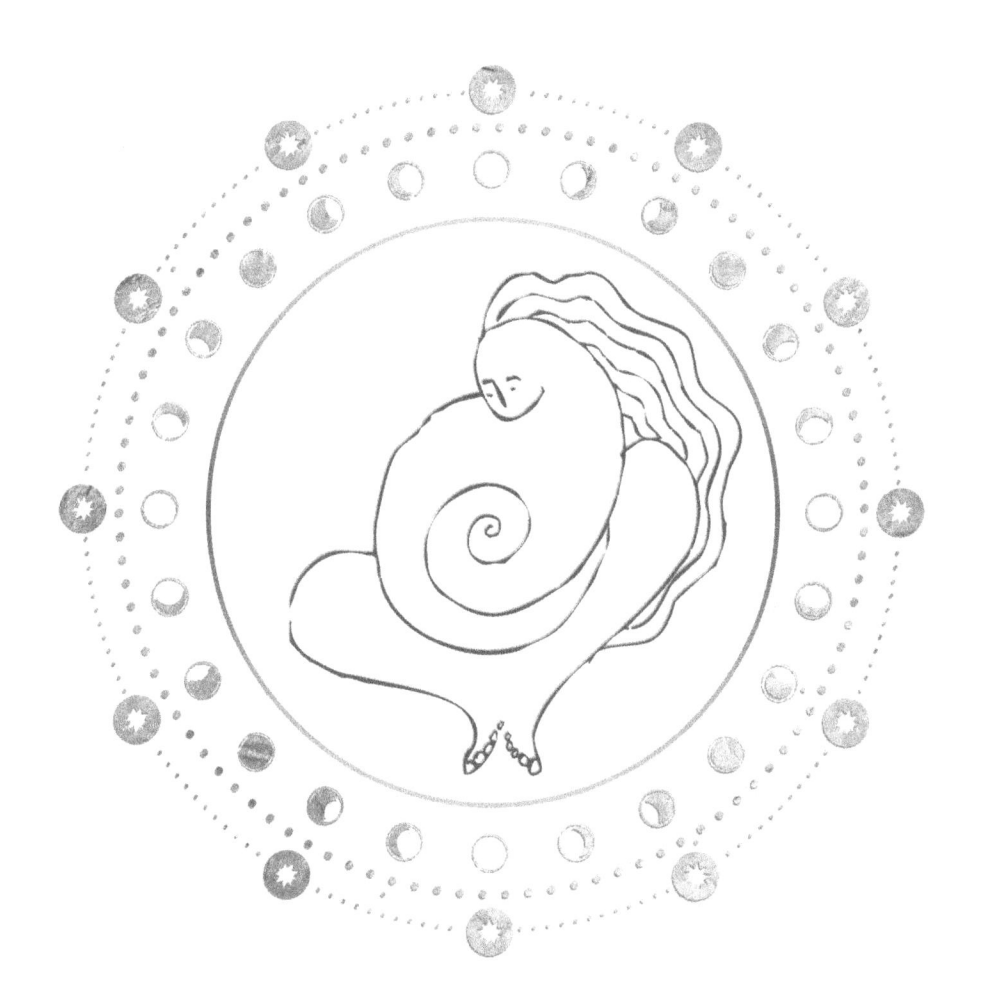

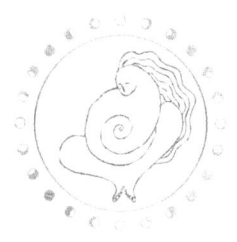

What have you been told or taught about what it is to be a woman, thinking back to the first messages you were given from your mother, father, friends and media?

Well, for me it's on many levels. I was born and bred in London. As I remember this, I can see myself as a girl, young black girl, dark skin with a blue dress. I loved that dress and American Tan tights – they were the closest you could get to my skin tone. I loved my American Tan tights! I had very short hair and was quite round. I remember very early on feeling really great about me and my American Tan tights. Many years later in my adult life I was quite upset when someone said to me, "Yeah, you only had your American Tan tights because they wouldn't acknowledge your skin tone."

So, we all had to wear the same thing. I thought, 'Oh, I really loved them.' It's interesting – it's best to be unaware sometimes as a child. So many things like that.

So, American Tan I loved, but suddenly they became a, 'No, you weren't acknowledged or recognised. That's all we got, that's all they'd give you.'

And then I can see me as a child with some other black friends. Do you remember ponchos?

Yes, I do. I had one.

They were big in the 1970s, so it must have been when I was at primary school. I was born in 1962, so yes the 70s. Me and my friends would put the ponchos on our head and go into the toilets by the sinks and we'd be singing. It was important to have the ponchos because it was like having long hair. So, the ponchos reflected being white, having long straight hair.

So, it is really interesting, you asking that question, because even though I was a child, it was innocent, but I look back and think, 'Oh god.' Like watching the Black and White Minstrel Show (UK Saturday night entertainment programme). Loving every part of it and not realising it's a representation of *you*. But I was watching these people dancing and just wanting to dance myself. Not even seeing them as blacked up. Actually, I think my parents did really well, because at no point did I think they represented me. Clearly, they were white people blacked up. I didn't see it as a reflection of our state. It wasn't anything to be considered. Not thinking any less of myself. But it was all the subtleties, all those subtleties.

And then in relation to a Catholic upbringing – I had a strict Catholic upbringing plus a strict Caribbean upbringing. It was a double whammy and then all the stuff that came with having a menstrual cycle in relation to those two upbringings. Everyone dreaded their period. I still have conversations with my cousins and we laugh that it was made to be such a disgusting thing. It was so horrible. Maybe I realise I'm sensitive. No, it *was* horrible.

I heard a story once, of someone who hid her used sanitary towels behind her family sofa. We were all made to feel so bad.

Who were you made to feel bad by?

My mother.

So, what sort of things was she saying to you? What were the messages she gave you?

You know, it's interesting, I can't remember her saying anything. But there must have been a real energy in the house for a young woman to want to hide her period, which I did.

What about your sisters? Did you talk to each other about your period?

My older sister was from the Caribbean, so I don't know what she was told. My mum would send us to buy sanitary towels. She was open about that. But it was all warped; there was a warped thing about it.

So, do you think that feeling was coming purely from what your mother wasn't saying to you? Or was it the mix of your mother and strict Catholic upbringing, being told women are sinful and the strict Caribbean upbringing telling you your blood was disgusting?

I don't know. I don't know what my mother was taught about it all. It's really interesting what the mind can do. Everyone at school hated having their period. It was disgusting to us all. There had been the whole sex education talk which was basically, when you start having periods you can get pregnant, so you'd better not do it. Catholic school – they were all up tight. I remember once in the sixth form we were all called to the hall. The priest was so red in the face and he was so furious, shouting at us about masturbation. And we were all thinking, 'Who was masturbating?'

How would he have known?

I know! He called us in and we had this huge lecture. I don't know what had happened or how he knew. So, there was a whole lot of stuff around sex that was warped too. It was all warped.

Take me back to the day you started bleeding and what you recall of that.

Well, we were always dreading that because of the dirtiness around it. It was all dirty. This was even at school. If someone had a period, all the girls in the playground would be saying, 'Urgh.'

Was it an all-girls school?

No, mixed. Mixed Catholic. The blood thing was all dirty. I remember starting my period and going to my mother and saying something like, 'I've started my period and I don't know what to do.'

I've got older sisters, so they would already have started their period by then, but there was no conversation around this, which is weird right? There were four women in the house, three men. So, I went to mum and remember feeling really afraid to tell her, there was so much fear around it. I went to her and she was furious at me and said,

"Go in the bathroom, have a wash, get clean, get the Dettol."

Dettol?

Dettol. 'Get the Dettol, go and have a clean.' I felt so ashamed, it was so painful. Then my mum sent someone to get the sanitary towels, my sister or my brother. Do you remember the Dr Whites towels? The big fat ones, there was nothing else available at the time, none of these slimline pads! These were thick and fat!

So, that was my welcome, made to feel disgusted in every way – 'Go and have a wash; use the Dettol.'

Can I ask, did you use the Dettol?

Yes, the Caribbeans were obsessed with Dettol and cleaning. In those days there weren't such things as a bidet, well we didn't have one. We filled an enamel potty, put Dettol in it and used it like a bidet. It was all about Dettol. I was talking about this, about the Dettol thing, because during the pandemic it's been said Dettol is the answer. We thought, 'Flipping Dettol, it still exists, such disgusting stuff!

So, then I had the most excruciating period pains, of course. I crawled on all fours in so much pain, every month until I had my first born. A friend said to me, "Your period pain will stop now, after you've given birth."

I thought, 'Oh it's worth getting pregnant and worth giving birth, to be released from this pain.'

I took lots of painkillers for the period pain, but in the end they didn't work. I remember being at a bus stop and my period starting and feeling like I was going to die.

It's interesting because when I started learning homeopathy, I thought to myself, 'Oh, that's why you had period pains.' It was all about a sense of shame, disgust, dirty, all that guilt, all that ugliness that bound the whole menstrual cycle. So actually, studying homeopathy was the best thing I ever did in relation to that.

When did that come into your life?

That came in after I decided to take a break from my dance company, to see what else there was for me. I was always into complementary medicine and ways of being. I was 40, perimenopausal and I was thinking, 'There must be something else I can do, it can't only be dance.' I decided to look into homeopathy, which I'd found out about through my son who had been diagnosed with potential asthma and not wanting to put him on steroids. I came home one afternoon and told my husband, "I've signed up for a four-year course."

You say you'd always used complementary medicines. How old were you when that came into your life?

It's interesting; throughout my dance training, so definitely in my twenties, early twenties. I look back and say to myself, 'You were always the person who found something complementary.' I didn't call them complementary at the time. They were just things that I came across, or these ways of being that I happened to find out about. Then I would go and explore them. I met a guy who, 'cracked your body,' or I went to a person who put needles in me! I still don't know how I ended up there. My first port of call was never a doctor. If I had an injury or something I would find myself having a conversation with someone who told me about an alternative. And then I'd tell everyone else about what I'd found.

Having discovered those things around the age of twenty, I'm interested to know if you looked for anything to help with your menstrual pain? You said earlier your pain went after the birth of your first child, so how old were you then?

I was thirty-two.

So, it was another twelve years in which you didn't discover anything to help the pain?

No, that's interesting. I don't know why. I did do herbs, but oh they were disgusting. I think maybe because it was all up in my head, I thought it was all physical. Actually, that's a weird thing to say. Let me start again. I think for me it was, if I had a bad shoulder, for example, or a sore knee, I knew it was related to my body. But I didn't have that connection with my period. It was just, this thing that I hated, that happened every single bloody month, forever and ever thereafter and wouldn't stop until I hit the Menopause. I thought I was always going to be in pain, more than suffer and I really hated it.

I remember you saying in the Menopause Wisdoms Circle, how when we did the Womb Meditation at the beginning, it felt to you like that was the first time you had connected to your womb. Do you think you disconnected from your womb when you started bleeding, or maybe even before, because you had been given such strong messages about your blood being disgusting?

Totally! I think probably before I started bleeding. I mean, for me it was, 'The womb?' Who speaks about a womb? No-one spoke about a womb. So, it was simple PERIODS – SEX – PREGNANCY. NO – NO – NO!

All disgusting, that's all I got from Catholic school, that's all I got from home. You have a period, you wash it away, with Dettol.

And then it seemed to me there were suddenly lots of pregnant teenagers and single mothers. I actually knew a lot of women who got pregnant in order to get a flat, so they could leave home. I remember going to the council once to ask to put my name on the list for a flat. The first question they asked was, 'Are you pregnant?'

So, you had very strong messages creating fear and shame, which clearly impacted on you physically and probably mind, body and spirit?

Yeah, definitely.

And those strong messages that, to be a woman was all about the blood, sex and pregnancy, again creating fear and shame. And, there's this deep disconnection to your womb you recognise?

Yeah.

So, when you became pregnant and had your first child (which requires sex and being pregnant!) what was your experience of that?

Well, being pregnant was *lovely*. Giving birth was hell, because labour pains were exactly the same as my period pains. Up until that point I was floating throughout. Before becoming pregnant I had already been made to feel disgusting because I had moved in with my boyfriend (who became my husband). I remember asking my mum, "Why is it all my sisters get invited to be godmothers for children, why do I never get asked?"

I remember her saying, "That's because you live in sin. No-one wants somebody who lives in sin to be a godparent to their child."

And that felt like the same energy as the fear and shame of my blood, of sex, of pregnancy.

So, in labour everything was really nice, waterbirth, (although I never actually made it into the water!) NCT (National Childbirth Trust), all floating and then the first labour pain and I thought, 'Shit, it's those period pains.' For nine months I hadn't had those pains. It took twenty-six hours to give birth. Everything went out of the window. I was back in the face of *that* pain. I remember thinking, 'No-one ever told me it was the same as period pain.' I was so freaked out. All my birth plans – out of the window because the pain brought me right back to deep fear. When I look back, I think no wonder it all took so long, my body must have felt me wanting to reverse the whole process. I didn't want to be there back in the pain. I think I was in shock being back in that pain.

How many children do you have?

Two – two boys.

What was the second birth like?

By then I knew about homeopathy. When I went into labour, I thought, 'Oh shit, damn, it's period pain again.' That's all I had in my head 'period pain.' Thank God I had homeopathy. The hospital wanted to induce me. I thought, 'You are not inducing me.' I had my homeopathy kit; I knew exactly what to take and when. I woke up in the morning with period pains, immediately, he was born in three and half hours.

There's a five-year gap between my boys. I needed that space to be brave enough to go there again. I had thought I was going to die from the pain because it was so intense with my first child's birth. I actually thought I was going to die. With my second child, it was brief, intense. I did throw those remedies down me. But unfortunately, it was the pain again and I had an epidural, which is why I have back pain. I just couldn't do it; I knew what the pain did to me.

Then, when I was thinking of having a third child, five years later, I thought, 'You can do this.' But there were two things, one was the pain, I thought, 'Will I die this time round?' Really ridiculous right? Will I die? The other thing was this, I had the strongest feeling I was going to give birth to a girl. I could *feel* a girl. Everything was about, 'There's a girl wanting to come.'

And what did that feeling bring to you?

Well, I went for a reading and the woman said, "You've got a girl around you. Why have you got a girl around you?"

I remember shaking and panicking, I thought, 'No.' Because I'd made a decision. I was worried that if I was to give birth to a girl, I might damage her, because of my mother – daughter 'no' relationship. I've never said this to anyone before, maybe one person, that, if I have a girl, based on the damage, the trauma, based on the unresolved mother/daughter stuff; it's possible, because it's so unresolved and I haven't done enough therapy on this, it's possible that I might repeat patterns. And I might hurt her. I don't ever want to do that to another female, so therefore no more babies. That was the decision and where it came from.

Recently talking about this, I have thought, she might have been just the thing to help me heal, but I couldn't have taken that chance. Now I could have a girl! So much has healed, I don't think I would repeat it. But back then I was convinced I would damage her, unintentionally, without knowing. And I could not do that to another female.

That's very powerful to make that choice. As I'm listening to that, Pearl, I'm interested to hear, how did all of that impact on you as you became perimenopausal? You said earlier you felt perimenopause arrive at age forty and when we chatted about this in the Menopause Wisdoms group, you described how you loved the Menopause, which is such a contrast to your previous initiations of menarche and motherhood.

Did you know what to expect of the Menopause and do you recall your mother's experience?

Black women don't do Menopause.

I've just made up that line! I'm laughing here, because

a) it's a generalisation and

b) it's not that they don't know what the Menopause is,

It's that their understanding is limited and stops with hot flushes. My cousins and I often laugh and say, 'What is the Menopause? Who does the Menopause?'

We recall our mothers, aunties and such, the older generation, for all the obvious reasons, having come over here to the UK and all the stuff they had to deal with. They didn't have time to be pussy footing around the Menopause. They all did the, 'What's the big deal?' To have the luxury of having a conversation about the Menopause? No! That thing that women do, 'Get on with it, it's going to pass soon, no matter.'

So, that's a great title for a book, '*Black Women Don't Do Menopause.*' That's a bloody good title!

I love that Pearl, yes, a great title for a book.

Before you go ahead and talk about how you knew about Menopause;

in relation to HRT, I just want to tell you that just the other day I read an article saying that yam is being prescribed now as an HRT.

Black women use yams as part of their staple diet, so they will have been benefiting during Menopause without knowing. Maybe that's why 'black women don't do Menopause.' Yams were an everyday thing. But I think it's true to say that generally speaking, black women don't do Menopause.

When I was studying homeopathy, they mentioned yams. I was, 'Oh my God,' because I stopped eating them when I was a dancer. I was being told I was too big, my thighs were too big, my black body wasn't acceptable. So, I stopped eating all those Caribbean starch-based food in the hope that my body would change and get closer to a white person (and that's another discussion!!!). So, I stopped eating that food.

But it was through homeopathy and I was being wowed by a whole new way of looking at health and wellbeing. And I was so inspired by the woman's cycle – how it's linked to the moon – I was so excited by the power. I even decided I should be going into schools to help young women, every bloody school, because of the crap they're taught. I thought every school needs someone to go in and celebrate the power of their cycle, the strength of what's coming. All my female friends had to live through me sharing everything I found out.

What age were you when this revelation of being cyclical came in?

I was nearly forty.

Ah, so that's leading up to you arriving at your perimenopause phase?

That's right.

So, just at the point you are beginning to embrace your cycle, embrace your blood, you're leading into the cessation of your menstrual cycle. I find this fascinating because it was exactly the same for me and a number of other women I have spoken with.

Wow, interesting.

For me, every decade, I have a sense of, 'Okay, watch out.' As I approach three years from being a decade older, things start to shift, everything begins shifting. I think, 'Oh, here we go, I'm going to make a change.'

So, homeopathy brought back the gift of my cycle. The way I studied homeopathy was very practical, so there was the homeopathy and everything else, the moons, the stars, the nutrition, the herbs and more, I loved it. I was thinking, 'Wow, am I really a woman?! What! Now I'm forty-one and I know that I ovulate from one ovary each month.' Which is why we have period pains one month and maybe not the next when we ovulate from the other ovary. So, then when I was working with women I would ask, "Do you have period pains every month?"

And they'd say, "No, it alternates."

And I was able to explain why to them – one ovary one month, the other ovary the next month. All this stuff that we are none the wiser to, I suddenly knew through homeopathy.

Oh, and the cleansing part of our menstrual cycle – wonderful! If we were to go back to the primal stuff of it, the Red Tents, the coming together. For frigs sake, we are so far removed from all that. I'm going to blame Christianity right now as I speak. I've just made that bit up, at this moment I think that is true.

In the Caribbean there were lots of Catholics. It's all Christianity; my mum was into all that.

So right. I thought I'm going to be prepared for this, the Menopause. I thought, it's going to come, I'm already going into that space, and I felt so fascinated by it all. I thought, 'I'm going to read books on the Menopause so I know everything about it, the perimenopause, Menopause.' I wanted to tell everybody about it, so that when I got there I'd be prepared, I'd know what to do. I read Leslie Kenton's book *Passage to Power*. Oh, that book was fabulous for me. She goes into the whole emotional, spiritual changes. I wanted everyone to read it! I felt, 'Wow, this is what's coming – freedom!'

And then...

I forgot that information. Clearly, I forgot, because what I expected wasn't what I experienced. I was in it before I realised. When I reached what she had been talking about, it was far more subtle. I thought I was going to have hot flushes, dry hair, falling hair, whatever, right away. But it wasn't like that for me. It was very slow, very subtle and although the flushes came, it was more of the emotional impact. I think it was because I had little ones as well. I think it was a few things. I had to stop dancing because I felt I had to find out what else there was for me. So, I was training to be this homeopath. Juggling house, home, study. So, the perimenopause sort of slithered in and before I knew it, I felt like everything was falling apart. *Everything* – it was *so* difficult.

I think I was fortunate because the only thing I had to deal with physically was the hot flushes. And once I'd worked out my homeopathic remedy, I could allow my body to do what it needed to do and then dissipate as soon as possible. My body was quite pure and clean because I'd never really taken pharmaceutical medication, other than painkillers for my period which I'd stopped a long time ago by this point. It was difficult for a few years and then I realised, 'Oh shit, you stupid cow! You're perimenopausal!' Then I got the book out and read it all over again as well as some Dr Christiane Northrup.

And that was interesting because I decided that Menopause was going to be my speciality in my homeopathic practice. I felt, every woman needs to realise the gift of Menopause. To 'Move to the Menopausal Beat.' And then someone asked me, "Is this it then Pearl? Is this what you are going to be focusing on?"

I started connecting with other menopausal people, specialists. And then I had a freak out moment and thought, 'No, this is pigeon-holing me.' I decided I didn't want to just be doing the Menopause.

It was actually about women empowerment; I mean Menopause is one super-duper part of our empowerment. But no. I didn't want to stop my creativity. Pearl is creative, always creating different things. I mean I love the Menopause. I loved working with menopausal women, I *loved* introducing them to the power of Menopause, becoming perimenopausal, even when they didn't even know they were perimenopausal. I'd go into my fury that so many women don't know about the perimenopause, they know the Menopause but not the build-up of perimenopause. I think that's shocking. I would suggest books they could read and give them remedies to support them hormonally.

The best thing that I loved about working with women who had not identified that perimenopause is part of the journey of their self-nurturing, was to let them know this was *their* time. I loved painting the picture of what it means, of helping their children to understand. To realise they had spent their life nurturing others and to know, 'Now this is *your* time!'

And I would talk about giving themselves permission to look to themselves, see who they are, what is their Truth, what is important to them. The perimenopause was bringing them into a corner and by the time they get to Menopause, if they had not taken those steps to nurture and take care of themselves, well then it grabs you until you look. You can't avoid it. This is one you can't avoid. If you do, if you try to, you're going to end up ill in some form.

I know it takes courage. Having come out the other end, it's the most powerful gift.

I have to say – the black approach, most black people in my life – our approach is different to the Western way. You remember I said black women don't do Menopause? I was talking with some friends they said, 'Oh god, yes, I remember that. I was so hot and sweaty.' And they walked around with wash rags to dry the sweat. They were all so full of drugs (HRT).

For me, it's all about choice. Choose what gives you peace of mind. If that's HRT, fine. But with drugs in their system, I know that they're not actually doing Menopause. They're doing the drug version of Menopause. Whereas for me, I did the herbal tinctures to allow my body to do what it needed to. I know from being on the Pill in my early twenties, my body was still clearing that drug. It never entirely leaves your body. However, if you don't *keep* putting drugs into your system, your body readjusts. But the impact on your hormonal system, taking the Pill, is huge.

So I guess for me, it was always about how I could help my body to continue to rebalance itself – mental, emotional, physical and spiritual. The hormonal experience was so brutal initially. That healing goes on. When I joined you in your Menopause Wisdoms Circle and you were talking about the womb, I thought, 'Wow, who talks about the womb?' It has been so long since I was pregnant and even thought about my womb. All that stuff that we as women learn about ourselves. We just don't talk with each other about our cycles.

I met a friend in town and she was so red in the face and she was dripping like mad. And she said she had just been in a meeting and was flushing.

She was so hot but thought she'd got away without anyone noticing her redness and sweating. She said she thought she had managed to cover it and no-one knew she was having a hot flush. I looked at her and thought, 'I'm not saying a word.' In my head I was thinking, 'You didn't get away with it!'

And the thing is, she shouldn't have to get away with it. Really, let's get into that space where she can say, 'Hang on a second,' and she does whatever it is she needs to do while she's experiencing her hot flush.

Yes. I've been in meetings and I've said

"Open the window, I'm having a hot flush!"

I tell them I need the window open, whether they're male or female in the room.

I think also, it's about our female hormones being our Truth. Our hormones are always helping us to be in our Truth, understand our Truth.

I love that. That's a very clear way of approaching the changes from both a physical and mental perspective.

And when we *know* that, it teaches us our cycle, no matter what stage of our life we are in. If we understand our cycle, our hormonal shifting, it's our Truth. It's showing up for yourself, giving yourself the messages. Your PMT (Pre-Menstrual Tension) might bring anger; it's showing you in that moment there's stuff that you've got to be angry about that you've been suppressing. And then our hormones say, no, you've got to look at that stuff.

Absolutely. I think there are many young women now who are working so incredibly with their cycle that I imagine their approach to Menopause will be different to our learnt perspective. Our generations attitude to our menstrual years has directly impacted on how we have approached our Menopause journey. All those PMT times when we were feeling anger, we suppressed those feelings because we were taught it isn't nice for girls or women to be angry or express anger. So, when we come to Menopause that anger has turned into rage. And then, if we don't give ourselves the opportunity to just take a moment and look at that rage, to ask, 'What is that rage about?' We turn immediately to suppressing our feelings with drugs.

Yes, suppressing. I asked a friend once if he remembered his mother wearing wigs. She was quite flamboyant and had a different wig for every occasion. Black women often wear wigs, but this was different. I never felt like I knew who I was going to meet. I remember she crashed into walls a lot. I said to my friend, "I bet she was menopausal at that time. I bet that was what was going on with her."

It was a time of women being given anti-depressants and our attitude was, 'Oh, she's going crazy.' But no, I think it was the Menopause. I really feel for those women.

Yes, my mum was given anti-depressants. I do think things are changing. Conversations about Menopause are coming into the mainstream. It's about bloody time of course. And I am aware there is still a tendency for those conversations to be about suppressing the symptoms. There is still a strong element of controlling the changes. My view is to seek out the support you need and let it all come up and out and explode in a safe space if needs be.

There's the nutrition side too. I mean, just eat yams in their natural state. Get off refined sugars, get off everything white, rice, bread, potatoes, because it all converts into sugar which increases your hot flushes. Alcohol too, it all converts to sugar. I don't do flushes anymore but if I eat lots of cake, like last week with so many birthdays, I can feel the heat rising in my body. I understand it's the sugar, so I then eat more green foods and get my body more alkaline as fast as possible. And I know if I carry on eating sugar foods, my hot flushes would be back.

Yes, I recognise that. I try not to eat a lot of sugar foods but I do eat some and for sure they exacerbate my hot flushes.

Yup, I have sugar in my diet too. I eat cake, I eat white pasta, white rice, white bread (not the squidgy type) and I'm aware of what it's doing in my body. I think everything in balance is best.

So, how do you feel about sex and your sexuality as a post-menopausal woman?

Well, it's really interesting. I am so over it. I feel 'enough already.' It takes too much energy. I really just like to cuddle instead. I have no need for sex. I feel like the odd one out with my friends. I have a friend who split from her partner because *he* wasn't wanting sex anymore. I know women

I've worked with who have lost their libido and I've recommended homeopathic remedies.

But I'm just so content, it just isn't important.

I have had a number of clients who have expressed the same and how it has caused problems in their relationship with their partner. It's caused a lot of issues. Some have been really drawn to celibacy and found reading about it and learning about it, that many people choose celibacy. That's very supportive to know. They had felt such shame for not wanting sex anymore, thinking something was wrong with them. Feeling like they were supposed to be sexual. Those voices are very strong, 'You're not normal. Shame on you.' But you know, it's just how they feel and that should be okay.

I feel very content. I've reconnected to who I am. I'm finding the balance.

I hear you, that's been my experience too. I've noticed that there's always talk of how we can all enjoy a full sex life into our 'old age' but there is never talk about how for many women during Menopause and post-menopause we no longer feel a need or desire to be sexual. There is definitely a stigma about not wanting sex and I agree with you, that often brings feelings of shame and guilt.

Yes, the message that there's something wrong with you if sex isn't on your radar is so strong. And of course if your partner does still want sex and you don't, it can cause such problems.

I have a friend who says there is such a hoo-ha between her and her husband. She doesn't want sex anymore, he does. She says it's her body, her choice. It's an ongoing journey. But she has said when she expresses to him, 'This is my body, my choice.' There is more of an understanding.

Okay, so finally. Do you feel that you do now have a connection to your womb and yoni?

It's interesting. I'd say, no more than I feel I have a connection to my knee or any other part of my body.

I feel like I've got more of a connection to my heart, that's what I'm focusing on. Heart is everything, because of my experience.

But not a disconnection anymore, you found the connection and it stayed?

Yes, it's no longer the 'disgusting, dirty' feeling. I'm not in that space anymore, not at all. But for me and my healing, it's about the heart. It's about love, love pouring right through me, all parts of me. For me to connect to that love and for other people to recognise that love, that's my focus. With that love flowing through me, it puts me at ease with all parts of me.

Do you feel that connection to your heart and what you've just described, has been a part of becoming a post-menopausal woman?

Post-menopausal, giving yourself permission, is the time to do that. That's what it is. It's opportunities to see things you may have not noticed before. We wake up from the drip, drip, drip, of the hormonal changes.

When we hear the word Menopause, we often think of getting old. I've never been bothered about getting older; black people don't have issue about our age. We always say it's a white person's thing, worrying about age. White people are obsessed with their age. We don't care, we don't think about that. There's more to think about than getting old.

So, for me, it's like, 'Oh my gosh,' – looking back at being menopausal, realising it was waking me up to all aspects of who I am, physically, emotionally and spiritually. We have to start working that out. When we hear the word Menopause, we have to ask, what does that bring up for me? What is it telling me? Are you learning, are you hiding? Are you pretending? I've heard women saying, 'It's all downhill now,' or 'It's the end.'

I flip that. I feel like it's uphill, like the sky's the limit. Thankfully, I had this understanding and I recognised the power and the gift of Menopause. I thought, 'I ain't messing around with that.' I'd been given a gift. You take that gift; you honour that gift. You allow that gift to teach you everything about you. It gives you a chance to take charge, take ownership and say, 'Sod everybody else and everything else.' Ask, 'Who is my version of me?' The Menopause gives us that permission because we go through so much; and if we allow ourselves, we are blessed by the gift. I understand this.

But there are far too many women who have no concept of this. So, it's really great there is more media attention and world Menopause Day. But I can sometimes find the media irritating because they often portray a one-sided version of what it is. They poopoo anything else that tells the truth and the power. They still talk about HRT and its benefits – and there are benefits, because for some, it is the answer. But I'm about choice. Share what other options there are. This one size fits all picture, it really irritates me.

There is a concert that I developed in my mind when I was thinking of working with a focus on Menopause. I imagined it taking place in Somerset House in London; a Menopause Concert. Everyone who comes would have a sash saying something like, 'Moving to My Menopausal Beat.' I'd create the whole performance with all different artists, singing, honouring the feminine, poetry. I thought, 'Flippin' 'eck, I can so see it all!'

I did do a 'Move to Your Menopausal Beat Day,' a day of getting women to dance. None of them knew anything about the perimenopause. So, they got dancing and I also had a friend who is a nurse and a homeopath and she talked about complementary ways to help them. I talked about the mind-body connection. I loved it.

I am still so passionate about it because of what it's given me.

And it's recognising the rocky road of it.

Yes, I think even when we have the insight of the alchemy of Menopause, there is no denying it can still be, as you say, 'a rocky road.' And that's such an important piece to express, to say, 'It's okay to be on a rocky road. It's okay to feel like you don't know who you are or what you're doing.'

Yes, exactly – it's transformation. We can choose to go to a therapist to transform what's going on right? And we can choose to go through the rocky road of it. The Menopause is your innate gift of transformation. You can choose to shut it down but it will make it more intense. It's potentially intense anyway, so you might as well let it open up for you. Pretending or denying doesn't work.

Menopause is an innate thing that we've been blessed to have. Unfortunately, the patriarchy killed it for us, so many women aren't open to it. Their life experiences prevent them from having these conversations because they are accused of being woo woo or off their heads, which is really sad. Being hormonally gaga is part of the process. We don't have to fear the gaga. We can help the gaga by balancing our hormones. The gaga, this too shall pass.

What we are doing, these conversations, are so essential.

I love that Pearl, "The gaga, this too shall pass!"

What a great place to end our conversation, thank you for your powerful insights, such a beautiful gift.

Reflective Questions

What resonated with you from Pearl's story?

What insights have you gleaned?

What is your biggest takeaway?

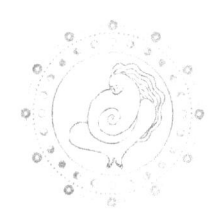

Part Three
SELF-CARE AND LOVE

Once again, I am imagining we are sitting together at the kitchen table. I wonder, what insights you have gleaned from reading the stories of our beautiful Menopause Wise Sisters?

How have their experiences supported you, activated you, triggered you or held you?

What will you do differently now you are walking your pathway to becoming Crone with a new narrative?

What ideas are bubbling in your creative juices to bring self-care and love into your life?

Who will you invite to walk this new pathway with you or who will you join to share your insights, wisdom, curiosities and experiences with?

In this section you will discover wellbeing practices to support your alchemical transformation to becoming Crone.

You may recall, in the Introduction, I said these are not prescriptive; they are suggestions and activators for you to try out and to guide you in creating your own practices, ritual and celebrations, as you gain confidence in your intuition and wisdom.

Let me remind you now, as I come to the end of sharing what I know, that you do not need to travel this journey alone. We sisters are holding each other, as we collectively co-create a new narrative for our Menopause initiation.

I would love to meet you and hear your wisdom and inquiries, so please, feel very welcome to join me for my monthly Menopause Wisdom online circle. You will be sitting with Menopause wise sisters, you will be heard, you will be witnessed, you will be held as you speak what needs to be spoken. We also rest in stillness together within a beautiful music soundscape creating space to dream, vision and dive deep into our innate knowing.

If you feel a calling to receive one to one support through your journey, you may also like to get in touch with me for a chat about my Wilding Retreats and Soulful Facilitation, online and in person.

There is beautiful alchemy in working together.

You may now also like to dive into those questions at the beginning of Part Two, to get your juices flowing. I suggest you begin with the womb meditation, just as Bev, Nicola, Sitali, Jenny, Louise, Maggie, Meg, Pearl, Sharie, Mia and Louisa did.

Imagine you are sitting in circle with them, with all our sisters wherever they may be.

Wishing you so much love,

Brier Heart

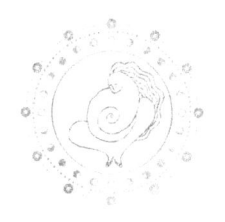

EXPLORING A NEW PERSPECTIVE

Try this exercise as a starting point to rewrite the narrative.

Take your time with this, be gentle with yourself if you cannot find the words to reshape the old stories or experiences straight away. The tales we have been told are powerful. But it is never too late to question and reframe old beliefs.

Create a peaceful space for yourself. Make sure you will not be disturbed. You may like to light a candle and play some gentle music.

Now, in your journal, make a list of all the symptoms and changes you are experiencing or have experienced in relation to The Menopause.

When your list is complete, put your pen and journal down.

Lie down or sit with your eyes closed for as long as need, with an internal focus on your list.

When you are ready to return to your list, take three deep breaths in through your nose and exhale out through your mouth, with a sigh or a sound.

On a clean page in your journal, list your symptoms again and your attitude toward them, leave a couple of lines clear beneath each one.

On the clear lines underneath each symptom and attitude listed, experiment with reshaping your response using different language.

Here are a couple of my own as examples:

Hot flushes. Embarrassing and inconvenient (old language).

Power surges. Clearing away old energy (reshaping language).

Insomnia. Frustrating, upsetting, exhausting.

Time to reflect. Journal writing. Time to be alone with a cup of tea in the peace and quiet of the night.

Exhaustion. Unable to function. Made me tearful and irritable.

Recognising my body needs to rest. Taking cat naps. Rescheduling or cancelling work or social commitments.

Rage. Unacceptable, dangerous.

A signal to explore my wounding. A prompt to seek out support in healing, to find a safe container in which to express your rage.

Continue in this way for as long as you need to.

The old messages have been with us for generations. Noticing them within is a powerful beginning. Where you are unable to find a new perspective right away, give yourself space and time, be gentle with yourself.

I suggest you return to your list when reflections bring new insights.

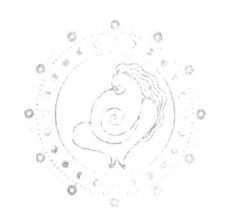

Journey to Your Ancestors - Calling in Your Crone Guide

I invite you to take a Journey to meet your ancestors and call upon the one who will help to support and guide you through your initiation.

Shamanic journeying was a constant practice throughout my transformation and for good reason. When we take a Shamanic Journey we deepen our relationship with Mother Earth, we open ourselves to realms beyond our 3D reality, we gift ourselves space to spend time with our spirit guides, power animals and angels'.

If this is your first journey, know that each of us experiences the process in our own unique way. Some of us see images, symbols or colour. Others hear sounds, voices, words. Or you may sense what you are being shown. Sometimes we experience them all. There is no right or wrong.

You will be journeying to the lower world, where we find our ancestors.

Create a warm, comfortable space in which you can lie down, or sit if you prefer.

Make sure you will not be disturbed. Have a scarf to put over your eyes. This helps us to separate from the middle world (our third dimensional realm).

Have your journal and pen close at hand for when you have finished your journey.

Read all the following instructions before you begin.

Set an intent for your journey. You are going to meet an ancestor who will guide you and support you through your transformation. You might say, 'I call upon my ancestor guide to be with me through my initiation.'

Once you are settled on your intent, repeat it a few times silently in your mind and then turn on the recording (link at bottom of page), after reading the following instructions.

When you are ready to begin, take three deep breaths all the way down into your womb as you prepare to journey to your ancestors.

You will then imagine you are standing or sitting at the base of a huge ancient oak tree. This is your threshold.

You will take in all the details of the tree, how she feels as you run your hand over her roots and trunk, her smell, her colours.

You will then feel yourself begin to flow into her roots. Begin your journey down, down, down, into the beautiful nourishing earth.

Down, down, down through her roots into the lower world.

When you arrive, all you need to do is allow what flows in.

Try not to push anything away, accept it all.

When you feel ready, call out for your ancestor, speaking your intention.

You will then reach, find, see, sense your ancestor.

Several may come to you. Welcome and greet them all and repeat your intention to find the ancestor who will guide and support you through your initiation.

Spend time with your ancestor. There is no need to rush. Be open to receive her messages of wisdom.

When you hear the call back on the drumming recording (3 x seven rapid beats), it is time to return.

Thank your guide for her wisdom and give her a gift before you say farewell and turn to leave.

Make your way back to the threshold and step over, back into this realm.

When you are back in your room, wiggle your fingers and toes, have a stretch, a yawn, open your eyes.

Note in your journal what arose for you and any messages or insights you received.

You can access a shamanic drumming recording via YouTube

I recommend the 15 minute Shamanic Journey by Michael Harner.

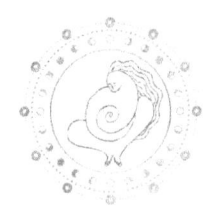

WOMB MEDITATION

Before you begin your womb meditation, read all of the following instructions to be clear of what to do and to prepare your space.

Have your journal and a pen close to hand.

This meditation is a gentle and powerful way to access your womb wisdom.

Your womb space (whether you have the physical organ or not) is your centre of creativity. It is a beautiful space of darkness. When we focus on our womb energy, we allow ourselves to dive into this darkness and connect to our innate creative wisdom. We invite in our flow of creativity, to then take out into the world if we so desire or hold within until we are ready to share what is shown to us.

Before you begin, switch off your phone and computer, make sure you will not be disturbed.

Choose a room that you will be comfortable in. If you choose to be seated, have a chair you can sit in for at least 20 minutes. If you are lying down, make a super comfy, warm nest for yourself.

You may like to light a candle and burn some essential oil.

Once you are comfortable, close your eyes and take a moment or two to settle into your space.

When you feel ready, bring your attention to your breath.

Allow your breath to slow and deepen.

You will notice your body beginning to relax.

Now place your hands over your womb centre, below your belly button and above your pubic bone.

When you feel ready, deepen your breath all the way down into your womb centre.

Feel your hands rise and fall with your breath.

Continue to breathe into your womb centre, slowly and with ease.

Now, imagine, sense or feel the beautiful darkness within your womb centre.

Pause here for a few minutes.

When you feel ready, silently in your mind, say "Hello" to your womb.

Pause here for several minutes.

Feel your hands rise and fall with your breath as you continue to breathe all the way down into your womb centre.

Continue to connect to your womb energy in this way for several more minutes.

Notice what arises.

When this feels complete, silently in your mind, thank your womb for her wisdom.

Begin to bring your focus back to your breath.

Make a sigh or sound as you exhale at least three times.

Allow your breath to return to its normal pace and rhythm.

Wiggle your fingers and toes.

Bring some movement into your body.

Open your eyes, stretch, have a yawn and smile.

Now take your journal and note down anything that arose while in meditation.

You may access a recording of this meditation on my website.
www.spiralsofwellbeing.co.uk/resource

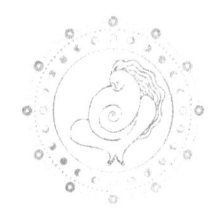

Womb Moon Wilding Dance

In 2013 I was processing Grief, my mum had passed and I was deep into the disintegration phase of my Menopause initiation. Feelings of rage and despair became powerful invitations to uncover and release patterns of behaviour which were clearly no longer serving me.

I also trained to be a Moon Mother during that year and my relationship with my womb energy and the Divine Feminine proved to be potent medicine for healing.

My body was calling out to me to find ways in which to release blocks in my physical and energetic bodies. Using my love of music and dancing, in addition to developing a relationship with my womb and the moon, I created a practice for myself which I continue to enjoy all these years later.

In moments when I feel *out of alignment* or when I simply feel an impulse to express joy and pleasure, because I am *in alignment*, I still find my Womb Moon Wilding Dance to be a beautiful act of Self Care and Love.

I make space and time to move, dance, swirl and twirl! I always begin by connecting to my womb energy, either through meditation or by simply saying "hello."

I make playlists of music which move me. Starting with slow ambient, the music gradually changes in rhythm and feeling, rising in energy to bring me to a trance state reaching a crescendo, in which I allow myself to be completely wild and free.

Then gradually the music returns to being gentle and flowing until my body is slowed to stillness.

I typically finish this practice lying on the floor for one or two tracks to cool my body and to begin to integrate what arose during the movement.

If you choose to try this practice, take your time first to be still with your intent. Ask your womb what it is that will activate what you need. Tune in to what you are feeling, name it if you can. Be aware of what phase the moon is in, notice how the phase impacts on and influences your movement and emotions.

I was often surprised at what I discovered when I began my womb moon dance. On some days I danced with my grief, on others I found joy led me. Each time is different, each time is healing.

As always, have your journal close by to record your experience.

This is my current playlist on Spotify:

Artist	Track	Album
Jami Seiber.	Benediction.	The Unspoken
Arooj Aftab.	Mohabbat.	Vulture Prince
Ganga Girl.	Mohan Meeting	Beats Around the Bush
Lula Cruza.	Cucarachero De Niceforo	A Guide to the Bird Song
Drumspyder.	Son – Maqsoum.	The Nekyia Vol 1.
Alex Reece.	Pulp Fiction.	Pulp Fiction

Bonobo Feat, Flynn.	Otomo.	Otomo
Makyo, Solace.	Naga. Tribal Dub Mix.	Revolution Rising
Maneesh De Moore.	Raindance.	Sadhana
Shaman's Dream.	Breath of Ma.	Prana Pulse
Nitin Sawhney.	Another Sky.	Immigrants
Malibu.	One Life.	One Life
MC Yogi.	Shanti. (Peace Out).	Elephant Power

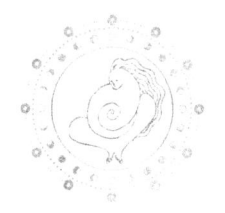

WOMB HEALING AND WOMB BLESSING

Soon after discovering I had a uterine fibroid and beginning my healing journey, I trained to become a Moon Mother with Miranda Gray.

What is a Moon Mother?

She is a woman who is called to connect to and work with the energy of her Womb Wisdom, the Divine Feminine, Sisterhood and Mother Earth.

A Womb Healing or Womb Blessing is for all women, with or without a womb or cycle, helping to heal and restore our female energies through Divine Feminine Love and Light. You can receive them in person or at a distance.

Becoming a Moon Mother gave me access to giving and receiving Womb Healing, Womb Blessings and holding the Worldwide Full Moon Womb Blessing Ceremony (five times a year). The energy from these practices is beautifully healing, potent and powerful. Women I have worked with have had life changing experiences; from becoming pregnant after a Blessing; painful menstruation becoming pain free after a Healing; and awakening to the beauty of being held in Sisterhood after a Worldwide Full Moon Ceremony.

If you would like to receive any of the above, or find more information about Miranda Gray's work, please go to:

https://www.spiralsofwellbeing.co.uk/resources

https:/mirandagray.co.uk/miranda-gray-resources.html

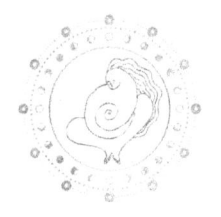

REWILDING WITH NATURE

Along with sisterhood, being in nature was beautiful, easeful and magical medicine for me while I journeyed my changes.

I live in rural West Wales where access to wild, free spaces is everywhere and for which I am deeply grateful every day.

But we do not have to live in the wild to find, connect to and benefit from nature's gifts. Wherever we are, we can find an opening to nurture and nourish ourselves in nature. Before coming here to rural life, I lived in Brixton. It had a busy city energy, but there were many beautiful, tranquil spaces within the frenetic vibration, such as parks, commons and woodland; which can be found in most urban and city areas.

We can too, create a connection to nature within our homes by tending to indoor plants, windowsill herbs, flowers or small shrubs on a balcony. Caring for these living organisms invites a reciprocal relationship of love and wellbeing.

Why not explore how you may bring the healing power of nature into your life?

Here are a few ideas to activate your creativity.

Take a walk in your local park, common or woodland. Find a spot in which to be still and silent. Hug a tree. Sit against a tree. Lie under a canopy of leaves and listen to birdsong and insects.

If you are walking along a busy street, tune in to what is growing through the cracks in the pavements or walls. Notice the insects attracted to the plant life.

If water calls to you, perhaps take a walk in the rain. Seek out fountains, a river or waterway.

Sit around a bonfire under a starlit sky. If fires are not possible, perhaps choose a full moon night to be outdoors and open to her energy. Or light a candle and gaze at the moon through an open window.

Weather permitting, stand barefoot on the earth. Have your feet hip width apart and planted firmly on the ground. Imagine you have strong, vibrant roots flowing down through your feet into Mother Earth. When you feel rooted to her energy, let your knees be soft and begin to gently shake from your ankles upward. Invite Mother Earth's energy to flow up through your feet all the way up into every part of your body. Continue to shake until you are ready to stand in stillness, feet still firmly anchored to the ground. Notice how you feel lovingly held by Mother Earth.

When you feel the need to retreat and be completely immersed in nature, honour your mind, body and spirit callings. Book some time away in the wildness of the countryside and/or coastline. Find a space in which you will feel held, perhaps where you can also receive eg, massage, energy healing, sound baths and meditation.

Please go to my website to explore what type of offerings you can access in retreat here at Spirals of Wellbeing. I look forward to welcoming you.

www.spiralsofwellbeing.co.uk/resources

Cycles Chart

FEMALE ARCHETYPES	LIFE CYCLE	SEASONS
MAIDEN	*Child* *Pre-Menarche*	*Spring*
MOTHER	*Post-Menarche* *Menstruating Years*	*Summer*
ENCHANTRESS	*Entering Menopause years* *Climactic Menopause years*	*Autumn*
CRONE	*Post-menopause*	*Winter*

White Moon MENSTRUAL CYCLE	Red Moon MENSTRUAL CYCLE	MOON PHASES	QUALITIES
Pre-Ovulation	Pre-menstrual	New Moon Waxing Moon	Innocence Playfulness Empathy Receptive Vulnerable Curiosity
Ovulation	Menstruation	Full Moon Waning Moon	Rebirth New life Natural Caretaker Creator Protector Responsible Commitment Compassionate Often Neglects self-care
Pre-Menstrual	Pre-Ovulation	Waning Moon Dark Moon	Impatience Setting boundaries Polarities of being Clearing Disintegration Fierceness Death Rage Grief Loss
Menstruation	Ovulation	Dark Moon New Moon Waxing Moon	Rebirth Reintegration Powerful Potent Creative Grace Stand in authority Knowledge Wisdom Worldliness Compassionate

The chart on the previous pages shows how each of the cycles I speak of throughout the book, relate to one another.

As we move through our changes and begin to emerge into new rhythms, noticing the qualities each cycle offers us can be invaluable to how we plan our day-to-day life.

I find it helpful to work and play according to the phases of the moon and seasons. For example, at the time of the dark moon, I am at my most creative, ideas emanate with ease. Inspiration is activated by this reflective phase.

I know that Spring is my time of feeling energised, nature is reflected in me, I am excited, playful and feel immensely free. I know I am able to get lots done in this season because my energy feels abundant.

I highly recommend you attune to how you feel within each moon phase and season.

How do they impact on your daily life?

Use your journal to record what you notice.

Red Moon Cycle - bleeding at the time of the full moon.

White Moon Cycle - bleeding at the time of the dark moon.

Of course, we may not flow with either a red or white moon cycle. There is no right or wrong. Your cycle is unique to you. Charting and noticing what changes there are within your cycle is the important piece, as this will enable you to respond with wisdom to your unique cyclical nature and energy shifts.

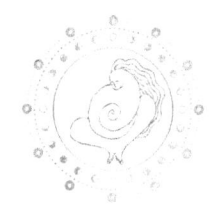

Deepen Your Connection with the Four Female Archetypes

You may remember I referred to the archetypes in Part One and they are mentioned too within the stories of some of the women. You will also see on the 'Cycle Chart' how the archetypes relate to our life cycle, menstrual cycle, the moon phases and the seasons. Each archetype provides us with insights into how we interact with the different energies within our cyclical nature.

I have loved calling in the energy of these female archetypes and finding different ways in which to connect with them. Below are some examples of how you may like to do this. Have fun with them, develop a relationship with them, listen to their wisdom.

Maiden. Her energy invites us to be playful, curious and adventurous. She calls to us to be unbound, to run and skip, to sing and holler, to laugh uncontrollably. The Maiden energy is rooted in her power of being a free spirit. She is confident, care-free, independent and an empath. She is unafraid in her vulnerability.

To connect to her energy, you may like to put on some lively music and dance with her, try different ways in how you move your body. You may be drawn to sing or make sounds, using your voice to express sheer joy in your Maiden energy.

Mother. Her energy invites us to connect to our creativity and to nurturing and nourishing ourselves and others. The Mother energy represents the caretaker, creatrix and protector. She is committed and responsible, but often neglects her own self-care. She also holds the energy of sensuality and sexuality.

How do you like to express your creative flow, your sexual and sensual energy? You may like to try using paints or crayons to visually express yourself, perhaps gathering things you find in nature and making an altar, writing your thoughts and ideas in a special journal, growing your own food and cooking sumptuous meals for yourself and others.

Explore and experiment with various ways to be creative. Perhaps call in your Maiden energy too to help you find unbound ways to be creative.

ENCHANTRESS. Her energy calls to us to set boundaries, to speak our Truth, to cut out the BS. She empowers us to stand in our sovereignty. She refuses to be silenced or shackled by external forces. The Enchantress represents a fierceness. She expresses the paradox of her emotional being, rage and joy, grief and bliss. She yearns for solitude and yet needs to be lovingly held.

You may like to try setting some boundaries! Ask the Enchantress where you are leaking energy and how you can address this. Call to her to help you weave empowered ways of being with your Enchantress energy. You may like to use this as an intent when you do the Womb meditation.

CRONE. Her energy shows us how to be still, to stop multi-tasking, to know we are worthy of time out and taking care of our needs. She invites us to focus on our inner world, to dream and to vision into what we wish to create for ourselves. The Crone archetype represents a woman of knowing and wisdom, expressed within the energy of grace, authority and worldliness. She understands the value of stillness, solitude and silence. Inner reflection comes naturally and with ease. She values our dream time, knowing important messages are revealed to us. She shows up exactly as she is.

Recording your dreams is a powerful way to develop your intuition. Dreams provide us with valuable insight, which if we pay attention to them offer profound wisdom. Keep your journal and pen by your bed and write your dreams down as soon as you wake up. You may also like to draw your dreams, to act them out through movement or dance, perhaps writing poetry.

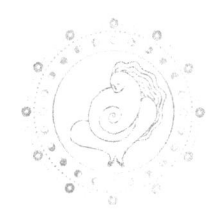

What are Feminine and Masculine Energetic Qualities?

There is a misconception that the feminine energetic qualities belong only to a woman and the masculine energetic qualities only to a man, when in fact, women and men have both the feminine and the masculine energetic qualities.

The imbalance many of us experience comes, in part, from being taught generation after generation that a woman must only demonstrate feminine qualities (which are often considered the weaker qualities), and men must only demonstrate the masculine qualities (which are often considered the stronger qualities).

I believe this is damaging to us all.

Finding a balance with these energies has been an interesting and long exploration for me. What I have come to realise, is that there is value in calling upon and connecting to, specific qualities in specific situations – that my feminine and masculine qualities are of equal value.

You may like to spend some time feeling into your feminine and masculine qualities.

Feminine Qualities

Compassion and care for others

Collaborative

Receptive   Grateful

Nurture

Interdependence

Relationship directed

Intuitive

Multi-Task

Temporal

Masculine Qualities

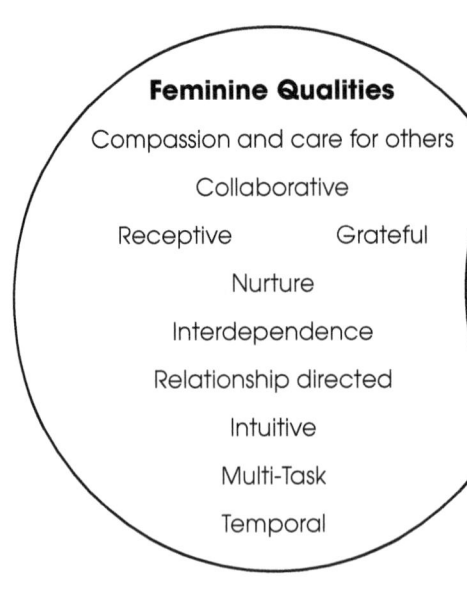

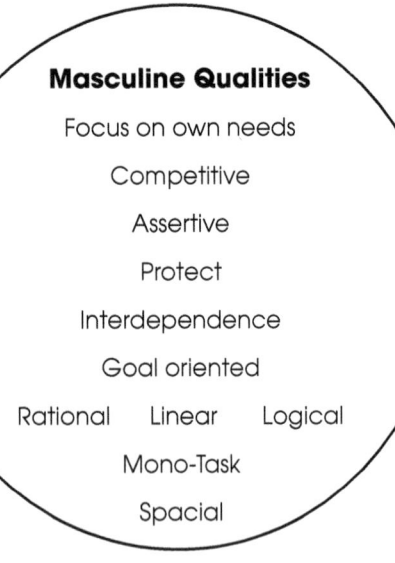

Focus on own needs

Competitive

Assertive

Protect

Interdependence

Goal oriented

Rational   Linear   Logical

Mono-Task

Spacial

How does each one feel in your body as you connect to it?

Are some qualities easier to access than others?

Which qualities are you resistant to?   How might you find balance?

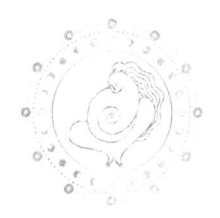

RECLAIMING YOUR MENARCHE RITUAL

As you know, the day of my menarche was not celebrated. You may remember from my story, how I shyly told my mum I had started my period. Her response was practical, showing me the drawer where the sanitary towels were kept.

I felt awkward, and a feeling of shame dropped in when she then warned me to 'be careful of boys now,' to hide my sanitary products from my brothers and dad and referred to my blood as 'The Curse'.

I was not told about the different phases of my cycle. No one suggested to journal how I felt throughout the month. I learnt along the way to record when my bleeding started each month but other than that, I paid no attention to the flow and fluctuations of my cycle.

My experience of menarche is not unusual, in all the years I have worked with women, not one has had a story of celebration about her menarche.

Reclaiming our menarche can be a powerful healing experience.

It was not until I was menopausal and began to question the stories I had been told about my menstrual blood being shameful, that I knew I wanted to re-shape and reclaim that moment. I did this through creating a ritual.

For my ritual I made a symbolic womb out of clay, from the land I live on. I wrote some words to honour my blood and the sacredness of my transition from girl to woman. I asked a trusted friend to witness me placing my clay womb into the stream on my land as I spoke my words, banged my drum and sang a song of love to my womb.

How would it feel for you to create a ritual in which to reclaim your menarche?

Think about how you enjoy expressing yourself, is it through dance, play, music, writing, art, being in nature?

You may like to call in your female archetypes to help you create healing magic with them.

Take your time to feel into what is right for you. You may choose to be outside for your ritual or you may prefer creating a quiet, undisturbed space in your home.

If it feels right for you, have a trusted friend to witness you in ritual. It is powerfully healing to be witnessed as we let go of old beliefs and invite in our new Truth.

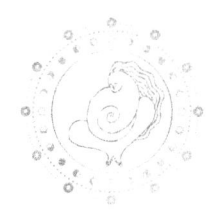

FEMININE RISING

During our collective experience of being in lockdown in 2020, I wrote a poem in response to what I felt was shifting at a global level. I asked my partner to write some music for the poem, feeling this would be powerful medicine to call in my feminine rising energy. I am pleased to share this with you here.

Create an uncluttered space in which you can move freely. Wear some comfortable clothing and have bare feet.

Have the recording of Feminine Rising ready to play.

Begin by standing with your feet, hip width apart, firmly on the ground. Then breathe deeply down into your womb centre, for as long as this feels good.

When you feel ready to move, press play, to begin the recording.

Listen to the words, feel the music.

Begin to shake or sway or quiver and shiver, whatever comes naturally. Start your movement from your ankles upwards, taking your time to feel each part of your body activated by your movement.

When your whole body is in motion, start to release each breath with a sigh or a sound, allowing whatever comes up and out.

Keep moving, keep breathing, allow it all. You do not need to stay standing. Often I will sink to my knees, or lie my whole body on the floor. Whatever calls to you, follow it. It is all perfect.

If the poem finishes before you have completed your moving and releasing, just carry on until you feel it is complete.

Finally, slow your movement, bring your breathing back to your usual pace and rhythm, until you are motionless.

If you are still standing, lie down where you will be comfortable.

Spend a few minutes in relaxation, then reach for your journal and pen to record what came up for you.

You can access the Feminine Rising recording via my website:

https://www.spiralsofwellbeing.co.uk/resources

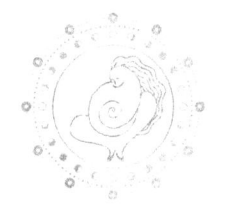

Dark Moon Dreaming

For many years now I have held Circle for women at the time of the Dark Moon. We come together to be still and silent, to journey, vision and dream into the beautiful space of darkness and to a gentle music soundscape. This offers rest, reflection and re-energising for the rising of the new waxing moon.

Mark in your diary when the next dark moon is. Plan ahead to have time and space in which to be with yourself.

On the day, create a nest to be comfortable in, turn off your phone.

Choose some gentle music, preferably with no lyric, to listen to while you dream into the darkness.

Have a scarf or piece of cloth to place over your eyes, turn lights off, blow out your candles!

When you feel ready, slow and deepen your breath.

As your breath deepens, become aware of the energy of the dark moon.

Stay with this focus for several minutes.

Now imagine, sense or feel the dark moon energy flowing down from above, down into your head, flowing down through your body, all the way down to your toes and out into the earth beneath you.

Pause here for several minutes.

Feel the darkness holding you, gently, lovingly.

Allow yourself to drift into dreaming or visioning while you rest with the energies of the dark moon and Mother Earth.

When you feel the experience is complete, take a few moments to come back into your room, wiggle your fingers and toes, have a stretch, a yawn, open your eyes and smile.

When you feel fully present, reach for your journal and pen.

What messages or insights did your dreams and visioning bring you?

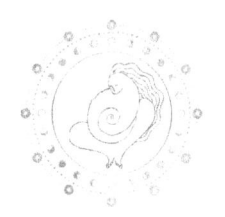

Creating an Altar to Honour Yourself as Crone

Creating an altar is a beautiful way to honour ourselves within the processes we are choosing for our wellbeing. It is a creative and nurturing act, aligning us to what feels important and nourishing at Soul level.

An altar invites us to bring focus to what is being called, and to bring stillness, silence and solitude, creating spaciousness in which to be peaceful.

You do not need to already be in your Crone phase to do this wellbeing ritual. Wherever you are in your initiation, it is a powerful process to honour what is coming, to begin to feel into your Crone energy, to call to her and seek her wisdom.

You may like to consider these questions before you create your altar.

- Where will you have your altar?
- What objects will you choose for your altar?
- How and why are they significant to your relationship with your Menopause journey as you become or are Crone?
- Find or make an object which reflects your feelings about your initiation to add to your altar.

When you feel your altar is complete, light a candle and stand or sit in front of it, say a few words in prayer or meditation to your Crone wisdom.

Ask her for her presence in your life as you navigate becoming or being Crone.

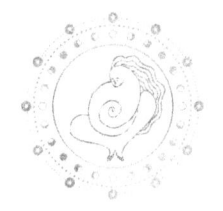

FURTHER EXPLORATION

I will leave you now with a simple reminder of the Self Care and Love practices our sisters of Menopause Wisdoms shared with us in their stories. I have no doubt that their individual experiences of finding what worked for them will have inspired you to further explore creating your own pathways to Self Care and Love.

Natural Medicine.

Herbal remedies, homeopathy, essential oils, massage, acupuncture.

Exercise.

Running, swimming, walking, dancing, yoga.

Spiritual/Soulful Medicine.

Meditation, breath work, voice work, poetry, journaling, being in Sisterhood.

Allopathic Medicine.

HRT.

Books.

Menopause Years. The Wild Woman Way by Susun S. Weed

Wild Power by Alexander Pope and Sjanie Hugo Wurlitzer

The Wisdom of Menopause/Women's Bodies Women's Wisdom by Dr Christiane Northrup

Red Moon by Miranda Gray

Code Red by Lisa Lister

The Great Cosmic Mother by Monica Sjöö

Gyn/Ecology by Mary Daly

The Female Eunuch by Germaine Greer

Heal Your Body by Louise Hay

Passage to Power by Leslie Kenton

Take off Your Armour and Have a Cup of Tea by Angie Northwood

ACKNOWLEDGEMENTS

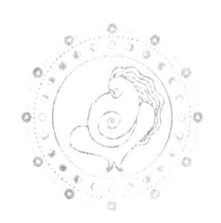

I would like to express huge thanks to my Unbound writing sisters in the Unbound Writing Mastermind group. The unconditional love, support, and wisdom within this circle of women has held me and guided me throughout the creation of this book.

Super special thanks to Nicola Humber, creator of the Unbound Writing Mastermind and the Unbound Press. She is a constant source of creativity and inspiration, playfulness and love, holding a powerful container for women to become their unbound self.

Eternal love to my husband who has made me laugh for over thirty years and who honours me and loves me as a Crone woman.

And finally, such deep gratitude to Sitali, Meg, Jenny, Nicola, Maggie, Bev, Louise, Mia, Sharie, Louisa and Pearl for gifting their Wild Wise Woman stories to us.